Emil Kleen

Carlsbad

A medico-practical guide

Emil Kleen

Carlsbad
A medico-practical guide

ISBN/EAN: 9783337412227

Printed in Europe, USA, Canada, Australia, Japan

Cover: Foto ©Lupo / pixelio.de

More available books at **www.hansebooks.com**

A MEDICO-PRACTICAL GUIDE

BY

EMIL KLEEN, M.D., Ph.D.
PRACTISING PHYSICIAN AT CARLSBAD

G. P. PUTNAM'S SONS

NEW YORK
27 West Twenty-third St.

LONDON
24 Bedford St., Strand

The Knickerbocker Press
1893

Electrotyped, Printed and Bound by
The Knickerbocker Press, New York
G. P. Putnam's Sons

PREFACE.

This book purposes to give the Anglo-American visitor to Carlsbad some information about his "cure," and to enable him, independently of local information, to make the best possible arrangements for himself in the place. I have tried to be as comprehensive and still to condense matters as much as possible. Purely scientific things are either entirely omitted or passed over in the most general way ; matters of mere local interest are also avoided or very briefly treated of, in order to facilitate the acquisition of important information. All of the little book is only—*mutatis mutandis*, and with some additions and alterations—in substance a repetition of what I wrote some eight years ago for my Scandinavian countrymen and patients, and has no other pretensions than to be what it calls itself : a guide (for the layman-patient) in Carlsbad. Having had to write in a foreign tongue I fear that I must apologize for the imperfections of style and language.

EMIL KLEEN, M.D., Ph D.,

Practising Physician at Carlsbad.

NEW YORK, February, 1893.

CONTENTS.

PAGE

WHO OUGHT AND WHO OUGHT NOT TO GO TO
    CARLSBAD.................................... 1
    Indications and contra-indications.

CARLSBAD'S THERAPEUTIC RESOURCES............... 9
    The Carlsbad-water and its products—The different
    springs—The baths—The hills and the "terrain-
    cure"—Massage and gymnastics—Physicians—Hy-
    gienic and dietetic discipline of the place.

THE DIET AND SOME OTHER MEDICAL TOPICS....... 37
    General dietetical rules—Dietetical rules for patients
    with ulcer of the stomach—Dilatation of the stomach
    —Gall-stones—Adiposity—Gout—Diabetes.

BEFORE AND AFTER THE CURE—THE NECESSARY TIME
    FOR A CARLSBAD CURE......................... 64

LIFE IN CARLSBAD................................. 67

THE CITY OF CARLSBAD............................ 70
    Geography—Distance from chief continental towns—
    Nature—Inhabitants—Visitors—Historic Notes.

PRICES AND MONEY............................... 76

ARRIVAL IN CARLSBAD AND CHOICE OF LODGINGS.... 77

REGULATIONS RESPECTING LODGINGS IN CARLSBAD... 82

HOTELS IN CARLSBAD............................. 86

COOK'S AGENCY IN CARLSBAD...................... 87

BANKS AND EXCHANGES........................... 87

POST, TELEGRAPH AND CUSTOM-HOUSE OFFICE....... 88

MAYER'S TOURIST OFFICE................................ 88

ULRICH AND GROSS' LUGGAGE EXPEDITION.......... 88

CHURCHES... 88

MUSIC.. 89

STADT-THEATER... 89

APOTHECARIES' STORES...................................... 89

MATTONI'S MINERAL-WATER STORE.................. 89

THE CARLSBAD-WATER FOR EXPORTATION........... 90

THE BURGOMASTER'S AND THE POLICE OFFICE....... 90

BEZIRKSHAUPTMANNSCHAFT............................. 90

TARIFF FOR THE BATHS.................................... 90

KUR- AND MUSIK-TAX...................................... 91

TARIFF FOR CARRIAGES.................................... 92

OMNIBUS-CARS AND THEIR TARIFFS.................... 93

DONKEY CARRIAGES, DONKEYS, AND THEIR TARIFFS.. 95

ROLLING-CHAIRS AND EXPRESSMEN AND THEIR TARIFFS 96

EXCURSIONS.. 96

Puppsche Allée, Kiesweg, Posthof, Freundschaftsaal, Kaiserpark—Dorotheenau, Sauerbrunnen, Schweitzer-hof, Schönbrunn — Hammer or Pirkenhammer— Hirschensprung — Ecce-Homo-Kapelle, Findlaters Tempel, Franz-Joseph's-Höhe, Belvedere, Friedrich-Wilhelm's-Platz—Aberg—Stephanplatz, Panorama, Camera Obscura, Dreikreutzberg, König-Otto-Höhe, Ewiges Leben, and Stephaniewarte—Wiesenthal—Dallwitz — Giesshübl-Puchstein — Engelhaus— Aich, Hans Heiling, Elbogen—Joachimsthal, Gottesgab, Sonnenwirbel.

WHO OUGHT AND WHO OUGHT NOT TO GO TO CARLSBAD?

CARLSBAD has acquired its unrivalled reputation chiefly by the therapeutic results won there in the treatment of the following diseases :

Chronic gastric catarrh.

The different forms of dyspepsia.

Ulcer of the stomach or of the duodenum.

Dilatation of the stomach (when not caused by cancer).

Chronic intestinal catarrh.

Hæmorrhoids and stasis in the portal-system.

Hyperæmia of the liver.

Enlargement of the liver.

Fatty liver.

Cirrhosis of the liver.

Gallstone.

Kidney-stone.

Catarrh in the pelvis of the kidney, or in the bladder.

The chronic interstitial inflammation of the kidney, or certain forms of those diseases which, by a common name, are called "Morbus Brighti."

Enlargement of the prostate.

I

Adiposity.

Gout.

Diabetes.

These were and are the distinctive "Carlsbad-diseases," "par excellence," which are considered especially to form indications for Carlsbad in its character as the first of alkaline-saline spas. To this list we are also entitled to add several names, partly of diseases which are in some cases treated at alkaline-saline as well as at other springs, partly of some affections which are not, *per se*, concerned with this kind of spas, but which nevertheless often are treated at Carlsbad, on account of its of late very much increased and better applied therapeutic resources, which resources have extended the indications for going there beyond the original (purely alkaline-saline) limits. Thus, certain forms of catarrh of the pharynx, larynx, and bronchi are not infrequently under treatment at Carlsbad. The enlargement of the spleen caused by malaria is considered as one of the "Carlsbad-diseases," and yearly takes thither a number of patients from southern countries (see p. 5). Persons suffering from any of the many forms of chronic inflammations, which by the public are called "rheumatism," often combine in Carlsbad the drinking of the water with the use of the baths, especially of the mud baths. This is also the case with persons carrying the residues of past acute inflammations (perityphlitis, peri- and para-metritis, joint affections, etc.). The splendid opportunities in Carlsbad for the modern "terrain-cure" (Oertel) are taken advantage of by many patients with weak hearts. Finally, many representatives of that numerous class of patients who suffer from neurasthenia, and especially from that group of symptoms which are known as neurasthenia gastrica or nervous dyspepsia, find in the quiet but pleasant life at the great Bohemian resort, in the baths, and in the healthy, bracing mountain air, a means to better their nervous condition ; and I venture to predict that this class of patients will hereafter very much increase, since the authorities have now resolved upon the building of a new bathing-house, with every modern balneo-technical means for complete cold-water-cure. To this I may in a passing way add that I have repeatedly found a moderate amount of the alkaline-saline water to have, *per se*, an excellent influence in cases which, by their character and the result of the usual tests (Leube's and Ewald's), have shown themselves to belong to the pure "nervous" dyspepsia.

Having so far completed the list of diseases which may take a patient to Carlsbad, I have some not unimportant remarks to add. I have named the different forms of dyspepsia without excepting those arising from or being complicated with anæmia—as some of my colleagues, especially among the elder members of the profession, would most decidedly expect me to do. This is done for reasons mentioned at length at the end of this chapter, supporting my opinion that the widely spread idea of anæmia forming a contra-indication against a cure in Carlsbad is an erroneous one. When I, with other authors, name the dilatation of the stomach among the Carlsbad-diseases, it is with the full acknowledgment that alkaline-saline waters have no influence on the dilatation, *per se*, whatever. But they act beneficially on the accompanying catarrh, and on the dyspepsia, and when combined with the other means of treatment (see p. 44), give good results. Habitual constipation is not especially named in the list, because the modern abdominal massage constitutes by far our best remedy against this complaint. A "cure" at Carlsbad combined with that treatment is excellent, and, for reasons obvious to any physician, better than a cure at home ; but a well performed mechanical treatment at home is better for habitual constipation than any cure at Carlsbad without such treatment. The catarrh of the colon with habitual diarrhœa is not among the enumerated diseases, because the warm astringent irrigation of the colon is a better means than anything else in those cases, which, it is needless to say, also do better in Carlsbad than at home, *if* the specific Carlsbad treatment is combined with the before-named irrigations.

Among the different forms of " Morbus Brighti," only the interstitial ones with few elements from the kidneys and a small amount of albumen in the urine, especially the "gouty kidney," do well in Carlsbad. The "parenchymatous" forms are, in many cases at least, not influenced at all by the alkaline-saline water—as I have had occasion to verify by careful investigations.

The patients with enlargement of the spleen from malaria or from typhoid derive benefit from the Carlsbad-water, but ought generally to combine the pure Carlsbad-cure with an iron-cure. I cannot participate in the opinion of those physicians who forbid patients taking simultaneously mineral waters of different kinds. I have, with many other physicians, repeatedly given the Levico or other iron waters (or artificial preparations) to patients taking the alkaline-saline waters (they take the last-named waters as usual, an hour before their breakfast, and the iron immediately after meals). I have never seen any special disadvantages arise from such a course ; on the contrary, the patients stand the iron better during a Carlsbad-cure than at other time, and I greatly prefer giving them both remedies simultaneously, than letting them first pass through a simple " Carlsbad-cure " and then giving them iron as an " after-cure."

It is self-evident that only those patients can derive any benefit from a cure in Carlsbad whose condition—whatever their disease may be—generally admits of improvement. Thus the cirrhosis of the liver does well in incipient cases, but when it is far advanced, when the patient suffers from a great amount of ascites and has reached the end of his strength, the waters will not do him much good, the journey might be dangerous to him, and he had better stay at home. What I have said about the cirrhosis of the liver also applies to the interstitial nephritis, i. e., the cirrhosis of the kidney in analogous stages. The lighter forms of diabetes undoubtedly derive benefit from the cure and many a diabetic makes Carlsbad his summer residence for a great part of his life. But when the disease is complicated with tuberculosis of the lungs, or when widely spread gangrene has set in. or when the diabetes has attacked a child which is rapidly sinking under the swift decomposition of the albumen of the organism, and whose urine shows the ominous claret-like reaction with perchloride of iron, etc., etc., a trip to Carlsbad will be of no use. The weak heart before a decided fatty degeneration has showed itself or even a heart with deficient mitral- or aortic-valves in certain stages or conditions is welcome to Carlsbad, but an advanced heart-disease forms a contra-indication against a cure there.

The patient always acts wisely in consulting, before he goes to Carlsbad, an experienced and disinterested physician, who alone can judge of the pros and cons in the individual case.

. . . . . .

The contra-indications which are generally pointed out against a cure in Carlsbad are :
Acute fevers and infections.
Advanced (atheromatous and other) diseases of
    the heart and arteries.
Far advanced anæmia.

Malignant tumors.

Tuberculosis and other infections.

Purulent processes of long duration and other states combined with great exhaustion and inanition.

Most central nervous diseases and developed mental diseases.

Advanced pregnancy.

To this enumeration I have also to add some remarks. I consider the contra-indication based upon anæmia to be scarcely valid, if any complication exists which indicates Carlsbad. In my opinion anæmia forms no contra-indication against a rational cure at Carlsbad, though it certainly forms one against the very irrational cure that formerly was given in that place. A past generation of physicians gave the waters in enormous quantities and imposed at the same time the most rigorous diet. The consequences were that all patients got more or less "pulled down" by the cure, and this was especially the case with anæmic patients. Thus arose the idea that Carlsbad is dangerous to anæmic people, which idea still has a strong hold upon many foreign physicians and laymen, and survives long after the nonsensical system, which gave birth to it, has been abandoned. I have treated many anæmic patients in Carlsbad (for dyspepsia or other troubles), and I think that my colleagues in the place will agree with me that the results of small quantities of Carlsbad-water, of a nourishing, easily digested diet, and of the simul-

taneous use of iron and other specific remedies
against anæmia are exceedingly satisfactory.

Another erroneous idea is very prevalent among
the public, viz., that every person who goes to
Carlsbad is bound to be thinner, when he leaves
the place, than at his arrival, and that, consequently,
very thin people ought never to go there. This
idea is also a ghost of the old day of starvation and
of enormous quantities of alkaline-saline water.
It is generally no difficult thing, even during a
Carlsbad-cure, through the usual dietetic means
to increase the weight of thin people—a statement
to the truth of which a great many former patients
may testify, who on leaving Carlsbad were con-
siderably stouter than on arriving there.

CARLSBAD'S THERAPEUTIC RESOURCES.

These resources are of many kinds, and, notwithstanding my full acknowledgment of the excellent qualities of the alkaline-saline waters, it is less on account of my own views than from a certain concession to prevailing opinion that I, among all these resources, name first the celebrated *Carlsbad-water.*

This water is practically a warm solution of sulphate of soda, bicarbonate of soda, and chloride of sodium,' and contains besides a certain quantity

---

[1] The same salts, though in different and less harmonious proportions, are found in the waters of Marienbad, Tarasp, and some few other less known European waters. Among the American waters (in Colorado and other places) which sometimes are given out to be similar to the Carlsbad-water, none can in justice be even compared to it. The unquestionably valuable Saratoga waters lack the sulphate of soda. As this little work goes to the press, I find, to my amazement, in a book on Saratoga of some scientific pretensions, a remark that the absence of sulphate of soda is a rather indifferent matter, and as a reason for this original opinion is given the (perfectly correct) statement that the pure sulphate of soda has long since ceased to be used. Why has it ceased to be used? Because it has been substituted by the much-used " crystallized Carlsbad-salt," the main bulk of the solid constituents of which is sulphate of soda.

TABLE SHOWING THE CONSTITUENT SALTS IN
GRAVITY, TEMPERATURE,

Main constituents are :	Elisabeth-quelle.	Markt-brunnen.	Kaiser-brunnen.
Sulphates of alkalies.......	25.609	25.674	25.207
Whereof sulphate of soda......	23.769	23.860	23.411
" " "potash....	1.840	1.814	1.796
Carbonate of soda.........	12.799	12.705	12.674
Chloride of sodium........	10.314	10.304	10.103
Carbonic acid } half combined	7.697	7.681	7.581
free..	6.085	5.557	5.641
Present in smaller quantity :			
Carbonate of lime..................	3.273	3.350	3.173
" " magnesia.............	1.642	1.634	1.602
" " lithium...............	0.121	0.123	0.121
" " strontium............	0.004	0.004	0.004
" protoxide of iron..........	0.026	0.006	0.029
" " " manganese..	0.002	0.002	0.002
Fluoride of sodium.................	0.057	0.051	0.053
Borate of soda.....................	0.030	0.040	0.056
Oxide of aluminium................	0.006	0.007	0.005
Silicic acid.......................	9.724	0.712	0.729

In all the springs, moreover, are found traces of Cæsium, Rubidium, Thal-
sub-

Total of solid constituents....	54.614	54.619	53.765
Specific gravity..............	1.00539	1.00537	1.00532
Temperature (Celsius and Fah-renheit)................	43 C.= 109 F.	44 C.= 111 F.	48.8 C.= 120 F.
Liters of water per minute.....	4.70	5.15	7.00

Parkquelle (40° C.) flows directly from Theresienbrunnen, Kaiser-Karl-
Krone, Spitalquelle, Hochbergerquelle, Bernhardsbrunnen, Kurhaus-
others. So is also the new Stephaniequelle, which, however, is only 71°

GRAMS OF THE SPRINGS, THEIR SPECIFIC AND QUANTITY OF WATER.

Mühl-brunnen	Schloss-brunnen.	Felsen-quelle.	Theresien-brunnen.	Neu-brunnen.	Sprudel.
25.799	25.088	25.588	25.479	25.493	25.915
23.911	23.158	23.785	23.774	23.654	24.053
1.883	1.930	1.803	1.905	1.839	1.862
12.790	12.279	12.836	12.624	12.910	12.980
10.288	10.047	10.314	10.278	10.309	10.418
7.672	7.493	7.704	7.584	7.627	7.761
5.169	5.822	4.653	5.100	4.372	1.898
3.266	3.337	3.293	3.277	3.287	3.214
1.613	1.615	1.615	1.577	1.592	1.665
0.118	0.136	0.116	0.113	0.113	0.123
0.004	0.004	0.003	0.003	0.004	0.004
0.028	0.001	0.026	0.017	0.026	0.030
trace	trace	0.002	0.002	trace	0.002
0.046	0.046	0.060	0.046	0.046	0.051
0.029	0.039	0.036	0.036	0.036	0.040
0.005	0.005	0.003	0.005	0.006	0.004
0.735	0.703	0.707	0.718	0.709	0.715

lium, Zinc, Arsenic, Antimonium, Selen, Formic acid, and other organic stances.

54.730	53.304	54.606	54.384	54.589	55.168
1.00532	1.00522	1.00540	1.00537	1.00534	1.00530
53 C.=	53.3 C.=	59.7 C.=	59.6 C.=	60.4 C.=	72.5 C.=
129 F.	130 F.	140 F.	139 F.	141 F.	162 F.
8.80	10.80	3.20	12.60	6.00	2315.00

Quelle (41° C) is chemically = the Marktbrunnen. Quelle zur Russischen quelle, and Hygieasquelle are not used for drinking, but are similar to the F , and contains more free carbonic acid than any of the other springs.

of free carbonic acid and of mineral salts of minor importance. The water reaches the surface of the earth in a great number of springs of different temperature, is entirely colorless, of 1.005 specific gravity—by evaporation an almost purely white residue of mineral salts is obtained. When the water reaches the open air in a very warm state (as *e. g.* in the Sprudel) it loses much of its free and a part of its combined carbonic acid. Some easily soluble bicarbonates are thus changed into less soluble carbonates and partly appear on the surface as a thin membrane.' To facilitate a review of the salts and of the different springs I give the above table, wherein the names of the. most important salts appear in larger type, and the names printed with smaller type represent salts of minor, or, in some cases, of no practical importance.²

' In this manner is formed the '' Sprudelstone," which, as a crust of several feet in thickness ('' Sprudelschale ") covers the fissures in the granite rocks, through which the water streams.   The Sprudelstone consists of 97 per cent. of carbonate of lime, and contains, in addition, phosphates and carbonates of magnesia, lithium, and strontium, iron salts, silicic acid, and water.   A part of the lower town of Carlsbad around the little river Tepl is built on the '' Sprudelschale."

² The Carlsbad-water has been analyzed a great number of times (Becher, Klaproth, Reuss, Berzelius, Steinmann, Pleisch, Wolf, Jahn, Göttl, Ragsky, Lerch).   The above table is arranged after the careful analysis of Prof. E. Ludwig and Dr. T. Mauthner, of Vienna, in 1879.   '

The temperature in some springs undergoes some changes from one year to another (*e. g.* the Mühlbrunnen). The above figures are from the official statements of 1886.

By glancing at the above table the reader will be able to verify the fact that the waters in all the different springs are, generally speaking, of the same kind, as far as the mineral salts are concerned. In all the springs we find to 10,000 parts of water 25 parts of alkaline sulphates, 12 parts of bicarbonate of soda, and 10 of chloride of sodium—even the other salts of minor importance are represented in nearly equal quantities. Only the free carbonic acid and the temperature of one spring vary greatly from those qualities of another.

These circumstances find their natural explanation in the fact that all the springs have their origin in the same source,[1] whence they, heated by

---

[1] One would suppose that this would be plain, at least to everybody who had ever been in Carlsbad ; that every one would, *a priori*, be inclined to believe in a common origin of several warm springs of the same peculiar taste appearing close together in a small valley, and that if other facts corroborated such a view it would spread irresistibly and would be quickly and universally adopted. But there are certain reasons for concealing the identity of the waters in the different springs, and the public possesses in an amazing degree a quality, which the greatest living surgeon once in a more frank than polite manner alluded to, in writing · "the average man is perfectly stupid in things belonging to nature." Thus must be explained the wonderful fact that a great many patients at Carlsbad believe that the springs have been collected together in the val-

the high temperature of the deeper strata and by chemical processes, are propelled to the surface by the constantly forming carbonic acid gas, losing, during their different passages, more or less of their warmth and their free carbonic acid. It has happened that when the Sprudel (which carries by far the greater mass of water) has broken out of its ordinary precincts ("Sprudelausbrüche") the water in other springs has diminished or they have ceased to flow altogether. When we consider this and the result of the analyses we must agree that the common origin of the Carlsbad-springs is as well proved as almost anything else in nature.

This little book is not the place in which to explain in detail the influence of the alkaline-saline water on the organism in general or on the different pathological processes, in the treatment of which it forms a more or less important item—an influence which is partly well known and demonstrated by scientific experiment and partly a matter of experience, for which the full and final explanation has still to be given. Yet it may be of some interest to the reader to know what with certainty can be said of the general and most important effects of its different constituents, wherefore I state them here in a passing way.

ley, only, as it were, for the greater comfort and convenience of mankind, that the Mühlbrunnen has no more to do with the Sprudel than the Potomac has to do with Niagara, and that the Carlsbad-springs are arranged in about the same manner as the different kinds of drinks in a modern saloon.

The sulphate of soda increases the muscular activity of the stomach and of the bowels (the peristaltic action), increases the secretion of the gall (without increasing its fixed constituents), diminishes the secretion of nitrogenous substances by the kidney̌s, and promotes the decomposition and consumption of fats and carbohydrates in the organism.

The bicarbonate of soda neutralizes in the stomach the acid gastric juice (and thereby for the moment annihilates digestion), by the combining of the sodium with the hydrochloric acid to form chloride of sodium ; it increases the secretion of gastric juice. The superfluous bicarbonate is unchanged absorbed in the blood, of which it is a most important ingredient, by maintaining its alkalescence, keeping a part of its albumen in solution, and partly carrying its carbonic acid. It plays an important *rôle* in the metamorphosis of substances necessary to life (metabolism), and especially contributes to oxydation and to the combustion of fat. It is secreted in the urine, the quantity of which it increases. It diminishes or neutralizes the urine's acid reaction, or may even, taken in larger quantities for a short while cause an alkaline reaction ; it may thus prevent the forming of uric acid concrements, and may possibly cause the disintegration of such concrements already formed. It has finally the quality of facilitating the elimination of catarrhal mucus from the mucous membranes.

The chloride of sodium, or common salt, is also

a very important ingredient of the blood and of all
tissues ; it is of especially great moment for the
solubility of some substances, and thereby for
almost every physical and for a great number of
chemical processes in the organism, and for the
whole metabolism or change of substances, both
as far as the building up or progressive, and the
excretory or regressive, part of it is concerned.   It
also increases the gastric juice both by its presence
in the stomach and its presence in the blood.

The free carbonic acid acts simultaneously on the
muscular and secretory activity of the stomach
and facilitates the resorption of the water.   At the
same time it makes the water more palatable and
acts in a sedative way on the sensitive nerves of
the stomach.   It increases the secretion of urine.
In such small quantities as in the Carlsbad-water
it has only a very slight and generally impercep-
tible effect on the central nervous system.

One may also concede some value to the carbonate of lime as neutralizing acids and as containing an important element for the building up and
maintaining of the bones ; the former of these
merits may also be ascribed to the other earthy
carbonates.   The iron- and manganese-salts are
present in very small quantity, but may be of some
value.   The remaining ingredients are, as far as I
can understand, either by their small quantity or
by their quality, worthless.

The high temperature of the water has its value
by promoting the resorption and by quieting the

peristaltic action (which is stimulated by the cold water). It has moreover its influence on the vaso-motor and other nervous systems and on the per-spiration.

From the analysis of the water in the different springs, we are justified in drawing at once an important conclusion : all the springs have in general the same pharmacodynamic qualities.[1] There is no special " gallstone-spring," no spring exclusively for dyspeptic troubles, for diabetics, etc., etc.

[1] When people, as sometimes happens, can believe the dif-ferent springs to be perfectly independent of each other, it is no wonder that they also believe the different springs to have entirely different pharmacodynamic qualities. This idea is always so formed that they believe the hotter, the noisier, and the bigger a spring is, the "stronger" must be its effect on their own organism. When they see the seething and puffing Sprudel throw its large mass of water several fathoms in the air, they not unnaturally but unconsciously transfer the impres-sion of its mechanical power to their imagination of what it may effect on their organism. The courageous and energetic patient expects that the Sprudel alone can help him, but that the Sprudel is positively certain to help almost anything. The more timid nature gets the idea that the Sprudel is entirely too strong for him, and some patients would consider it very little short of murder in the physician to send them to that formidable spring. When these patients see the Kaiser-Karl-Quelle silently send down its scanty little jet in the stone-basin, they despise the spring as "one of the very weakest of the whole number" But the Sprudel and the Kaiser-Karl-Quelle contain very much the same kind of water ; the lat-ter spring is only cooler and has a greater quantity of free carbonic acid.

2

"Is it then an indifferent matter from what spring I drink ?" asks the reader.

No ! Passing over the generally unimportant difference in the quantity of free carbonic acid, the temperature is of great moment and principally decides what spring is best adapted to any special case. In general the colder water is more slowly absorbed, augments more the peristaltic actions of the bowels and (contrary to the idea of most inexperienced patients) is more aperient than the warmer. The different temperature acts differently on the vasomotor system and for some people there are contra-indications against any high temperature, a fact which may be of great importance —it being even dangerous for them to drink much hot water. When the spring has been determined and used some time, changes may arise which make another spring more suitable or necessary, and only a very small number of patients use the same spring the whole time.

How much water ought to be drunk is also an important question, which can only be decided in the special case, and for which no general rules are sufficient. The rational quantity changes according to the disease, the age, constitution, and condition of the patient. The full-grown individual can drink more than the youth or the child, the plethoric or fat more than the anæmic or thin, the patient suffering from a gallstone must—*ceteris paribus*—drink more than the one who suffers from an ulcer of the stomach, a dyspepsia, or a gastric catarrh, etc., etc. The modern treatment only allows of moderate quantities ; a great many patients only drink one or two glasses (210 *c.c.* each), the majority do not exceed four, very few (and scarcely any with a physician's permission) drink more than six glasses.

The great majority of patients only drink in the morning before breakfast, during which time the springs are visited from as early as five and until nine o'clock. Some patients also drink before dinner and before supper, and I think this method might reasonably be more often adopted than it is. A patient suffering from (a beginning or developed) dilatation of the stomach ought never to drink at once but small quantities of water (larger ones contributing to increase the dilatation), and may take his allowance of water at different times of the day. The ulcer-stomach patients also ought to avoid distending their stomach and may derive great benefit from frequently diminishing the often too great acidity of their gastric juice by the water. In other cases again there may be distinct indications for taking larger quantity of water but inability to take any great quantity at once, and such patients also must drink several times a day.

The drinking is done out of specially graduated glasses (sold in the vicinity of the springs), which generally contain 210 cub. centimetres of water. The patient must drink slowly and let at least one quarter of an hour, but generally a longer time, pass after each glass. Some people drink, out of an

unnecessary anxiety for their teeth, through glass
tubes, which prevents them from drinking too
quickly and is not amiss—for those who sell the
tubes. An hour must pass between the last glass
and the breakfast—the gastric juice being unable
to digest immediately after drinking.

Most people like the Carlsbad-water, and some
people, who come for many years to the place, ac-
quire a longing for it. To others it seems insipid,
and some few persons after a time get an aversion
to it. It is sometimes, by German authors, compared in taste to a thin soup—a comparison which
to me (who like almost everything in Germany except the soups) seems unjust to the Carlsbad-water.
After drinking several glasses of the water one
generally feels the warmth spreading and the per-
spiration increasing. The secretion of saliva also generally increases in a distinct manner, perceptible in
a pleasant way to the usually dry-mouthed diabetic
patients. There is often, for a longer or shorter
period, an increase of appetite, which sometimes
keeps on during the whole "cure," but sometimes
subsides after a while to the habitual state. The
secretion of urine increases, micturition becomes
more frequent, eventually uric acid deposits disappear, and the urine becomes thinner and clear. The
water is slightly but generally very slightly aperient
when taken cold or moderately warm ; when hot it
has not unfrequently a contrary effect. The excre-
ments are generally moderately loose, and have
often a very dark color chiefly due to sulphide of

iron formed during the passage through the bowels.
During the drinking period in the morning people
with weak heads or not very strong circulation
often feel some giddiness. Small troubles of different kinds from the digestive organs are not unfre-
quent during the cure ; nervous patients often feel
various little symptoms from their nervous system ;
and though many patients never feel as well as
they do in Carlsbad, others feel generally better
after than during the actual period of the cure.

I give some notes on the different springs :

The Sprudel is in fact a collection of springs on the right
shore and in the bottom of the river Tepl (in the midst of the
town opposite the " Markt "), and forms the main outlet of the
alkaline-saline water. The " Springer," of pre-historic fame,
which presents a rather imposing spectacle, *à la Geysér*, is,
since 1879, surrounded by a magnificent iron building (in
which an orchestra plays every morning from 8 to 9 during
the season). The Sprudel is the most fashionable of all the
springs, and enjoys a great, though sometimes, as we have
already stated, a rather absurd confidence from the public.

Bernhardsbrunnen is situated in the Mühlbrunn-colonnade, was conveyed in pipes in 1870 ; it is comparatively
little used for drinking purposes.

Neubrunnen is also situated in the Mühlbrunn-colonnade,
was conveyed in pipes in 1847, has been very fashionable, and
is still very much used.

Theresienbrunnen, on the slope of the Schlossberg in an
upper part of the Mühlbrunn-colonnade (stairs lead up to it
from the lower part of the same colonnade), was conveyed in
pipes in 1762, and is visited every morning by a not inconsiderable number of patients.

Felsenquelle, just north of the Mühlbrunn-colonnade,
was not known until 1844, but is now very much frequented.

Schlossbrunnen, on the Schlossberg, was supplied with pipes in 1797, disappeared in 1809, and appeared again in 1823. Contains more free carbonic acid than any other spring except Elisabethquelle and Stephaniequelle, and is very fashionable.

Mühlbrunnen, in the colonnade to which it has given its name, was conveyed in pipes in 1711, is immensely fashionable, especially since the colonnade was built in 1878 (at a cost of 680,000 fl.) and since an orchestra plays there every morning during the season. [It has of late become somewhat cooler and is now some degrees lower in temperature than the above table indicates.]

Kaiserbrunnen, in the "Militairbadehaus," with an entrance from the Stadtpark, began its history in 1851, is as good as the other springs, with about the same temperature as the Mühlbrunnen, and more advantageous to people who dislike the throng at this spring.

Elisabethquelle, in the Mühlbrunn-colonnade, was conveyed in pipes in 1875, contains more free carbonic acid than any other well except the Stephaniequelle.

Marktbrunnen, close to the Marktplatz, was led into tubes in 1838, and is the most fashionable of the cooler wells.

Kaiser-Karl-Quelle, in the same wooden building which contains the Marktbrunnen, was conveyed in pipes in 1871, and has the advantage of never being crowded.

Parkquelle is the water from the Theresienbrunnen, conveyed in pipes to the Stadtpark, and has the same advantage as the Kaiser-Karl-Quelle.

Stephanie-Quelle, at Dorotheenau near Schönbrunn, south from the town, was supplied with pipes in 1887, contains the same salts as the other alkaline-saline springs and more free carbonic acid ; it is seldom used.

Quelle zur russischen Krone, Spital-Quelle, Hochbergerquelle, and **Kurhausbrunnen** are not generally used for drinking purposes.

The above-named springs are all of the alkaline-saline kind and carry what is generally called Carlsbad-water.

From the Carlsbad-water some derivatives are formed, viz.:

The Crystallized Carlsbad- or Sprudel-salt

contains 37.695 per cent. of sulphate of soda, 5.997 per cent. of carbonate of soda, 0.397 per cent. of chloride of sodium, traces of sulphate of potash, and 54.520 per cent. of water of crystallization. It thus consists chiefly of sulphate of soda, and is used all over the world as a substitute for that salt. By adding a certain proportion of the crystallized Carlsbad-salt to the Carlsbad-water, one gets a water very like the Marienbad-water, and acting more strongly as an aperient than the Carlsbad-water. The little packets of five grams each of the salt under discussion, which are sold in large quantities by the apothecaries, are especially in demand by fat and by constipated patients, who add one packet to the first or to several of their glasses in the morning. At the same time I mention this, I think it necessary to remark that the prolonged use of the cathartics of any kind whatever, for habitual constipation, is scarcely to be recommended. I have already stated that this common complaint is far better treated by external mechanical means than by internal chemical remedies, which never go to the root of the evil, and the effects of which cease as soon as the drugs or salts are discontinued.

The Pulverized Carlsbad- or Sprudel-salt (formerly Quellsalt) resembles, more than the crystallized salt, the mass of salts in the Carlsbad-

water, and contains 41.62 per cent. of the sulphate
of soda, 36.11 per cent. of the carbonate of soda,
18.19 per cent. of chloride of sodium, and small
quantities of the other salts of the Carlsbad-waters.
A teaspoonful of this salt in a glass of ordinary
water gives a solution which is very similar to the
Carlsbad-water.

The Carlsbad-Sprudel-Losenges are prepared from the
last-named salt, and are used as a remedy against hyper-
acidity of the stomach.

The Carlsbad-Sprudel-Lye is obtained by the fabrica-
tion of the crystallized Sprudel-salt, and is used as an addition
to the baths.

The Carlsbad-Sprudel-Soap is prepared from the lye and
cocoa-nut oil.

.   .   .   .   .

Besides the celebrated and valuable alkaline-
saline water we find in Carlsbad and in its neighborhood some other mineral waters of different
kinds and merits.

The Sauerbrunnen hinter der Dorotheenau—a water
containing free carbonic acid and small quantities of bicarbonates ; it varies in temperature from 9–15° C., and is used
for drinking and bathing purposes. There is another such
spring under the "Cambridge-Säule," and still another in the
house No. 232 on the Jacobsberg.

The chalybeate spring (Eisenquelle) at Wiesenthal
is used for baths.

Der rothe Säuerling at Drahowitz is also a chalybeate
spring.

, Of far greater value and importance than any of
these last-named waters are the **Giesshübler** and

the **Krondorfer,** which are both natural mineral
waters from the neighborhood of Carlsbad, and
contain carbonates and free carbonic acid ; they
are to the taste of many persons the very best
table-waters. They are all the more acceptable,
as the drinking-water from the pipes in Carlsbad
cannot be recommended.

.   .   .   .   .   .

Carlsbad was once upon a time only a bathing
place. Both its German name and its Czech name
(*Vary* = *Warmbath*) remind us of that time, and
it was not until the 16th century that the great
curative effects of the waters taken internally were
discovered.   After this discovery **the baths** were
for a time entirely forsaken. They are now looked
upon with favor again, though they play only an
accessory *rôle* in the treatment of the original
" Carlsbad-diseases."

But, as I have already remarked, Carlsbad has
of late much increased its therapeutic resources
to meet more numerous needs, and it can now no
longer be considered to be *only* an alkaline-saline
spa, though it still retains, undisputedly, the first
rank among such spas.   Thus, we will find in
Carlsbad (from next year on) such an array of
different balneo-technical contrivances as will
scarcely be equalled by any other health-resort in
Europe or America.   We thus name :

The mineral bath (in the "Kurhaus," the
"Neubad," the "Sprudel-bad," or the "Mühlbad ")
which is given with the alkaline-saline water, gen-

erally used moderately warm, of 28–30° Réaumur
(this thermometer is used in Carlsbad), for ¼–½
hour, with or without a cold douche afterwards of
rarely more than a minute's duration.

The mud- [1] **or peat-bath** (in the " Kurhaus "
and the " Neubad "), prepared by the mineral
water and by heated mud, and used either as a
whole bath of about 30° Réaumur [1] and 10–20–30
minutes' duration, or as a local bath, in which latter
case I sometimes order it to be as hot as the patient
can bear it, and extend the duration of it from half
an hour to an hour.

The Russian or hot steam-bath (in the
" Kurhaus ") consists of the patient submitting his
naked body to the influence of hot steam for 10–25
minutes, beginning with a lower temperature (30°
Réaumur) and successively arriving at the highest
one (40° Réaumur, or sometimes more). After this

---

[1] The mud contains sulphates of alkalies and of earths,
iron- and manganese salts, silicic acid and some salts thereof,
carbon, resinous substances, gallo-tannic acid, and remnants of
plants.   Many laymen and some physicians believe in the effi-
cacy of adding Sprudel-soap or certain salts to these baths.
I have sometimes heard patients express a hair-raising doubt
whether the same mud-bath may not be used more than once.
This is a perfectly false alarm ; the mud is only used once—a
fact that can easily be observed by the patients themselves.—
The city of Carlsbad owns an inexhaustible supply of it in a
moor near Franzensbad, whence it is transported by rail-
way to Carlsbad.   During the mud-bath, as in general during
hot baths, the patient may with some advantage keep a towel
dipped in cold water on his head.

the patient takes a douche slowly descending in temperature, and sometimes a dip in cold water ; finally he rests for a while on a sofa, covered with a blanket.

The Turkish or hot air-bath [1] (in the new but still unnamed bath-house near the " Kurhaus ") is not unlike the Russian bath, but it consists in hot air instead of steam, and in many places includes a *séance* of general massage.

The cold-water-cure establishment in the (yet unnamed) bath-house in the Marienbaderstrasse will offer all the items of the cold-water cure. These are chiefly : (1.) The different forms of cold baths, which always are of short duration ; (2) the wet packs, which combine the effects of a cold bath with those of a moderately warm one, and consists of wrapping up the patient in a linen sheet, wet with cold water, and covering him with blankets for half an hour or more; and (3) finally

---

[1] My enumerating among the therapeutic resources of Carlsbad the Turkish and the electric baths, and the cold-water-cure-establishment is an anticipation, but, nevertheless, a justified one. The authorities have resolved upon the building of a new house near the " Kurhaus," which will contain Turkish baths (hitherto not to be found in Carlsbad) and Russian baths (which are now in the " Kurhaus "). The building of a new bath-house in the Marienbaderstrasse has also been determined upon ; it will contain everything belonging to a complete cold-water-cure, some electrical bath-rooms will leave nothing to desire in point of modern balneo-technical arrangements, and will prove a very valuable addition to the resources of Carlsbad.

douches of different descriptions.—In the same house will be found some rooms for—

The electric bath, generally taken moderately warm and similar to any other moderately warm bath, but with an electric current passing through the whole length of the bath.

The steel or iron bath (in the Wiesenthal) is taken in moderately warm water, and is like the ordinary tepid bath.

The carbonic acid or acidulous bath (in the Dorotheenau) is also distinguished from the tepid bath by the greater amount of free carbonic acid in the water.   Finally we have

The river bath in the swimming school at Eger, but rarely used by the visitor-patient in Carlsbad.

It does not lie within the scope of this little book to give an account of our present (still rather imperfect) knowledge of the physiological effects of different kinds of baths upon the skin, the vaso-motor nerves and the nervous system in general, on the intra-arterial pressure, the heart, the kid-neys, and other internal organs, and the metamor-phosis of substances (metabolism).   Still I think it not out of place to submit to the reader a few scattered remarks touching upon this subject. First, I wish it to be understood that the baths act much less by their chemical than by their physical qualities.   The moderately warm " mineral " bath used in Carlsbad has very much the same (" seda-tive" and other) effects as a bath of the same temperature and duration in ordinary water. [The carbonate of soda makes it more effective as a cleansing bath; the chloride of sodium may form a contra-indication against the mineral bath in some cases of skin-diseases; the effects of the sulphate of soda have, if they exist for the bath, never been demonstrated; the free carbonic acid is present in too small a quantity to be of any importance whatever].—The mud-baths have without doubt their chief, (and a very great,) importance in promoting the resorption of the products of acute or chronic inflammations, as exudations in and around the joints, in the pelvis or abdominal cavity, "rheumatic" infiltrations in the muscles, etc.; they ought in most of these cases to be combined with (the still more effective) massage.—The Russian steam- and the Turkish hot-air bath have both a very strong effect on perspiration and on the metamorphosis of substances, but should be used only by persons who are, at least, fairly strong and healthy. —Every one knows the invigorating influence and the great importance which a cold-water-cure has in nervous disorders of many kinds and especially in that trouble (now so prevalent) which is called "neurasthenia," or (with a somewhat free translation) general nervousness.—The same beneficial influence is ascribed to electric baths.—The acidulous bath is also considered, by virtue of the millions ot little bubbles ot free carbonic acid and their action upon the skin, to have a bracing or stimulating effect.—The baths in chalybeate waters

are, in my opinion, of the same value as equally
warm baths in ordinary waters, be it said, however,
with full respect for the opinion of others who on
account of the (not absorbed) iron ascribe to them
a special "tonic "effect.—The cold douche is of great
value on account of its effects on the nerves and especially by its effects on the vasomotor nerves, which
bring about a contraction in the peripheral vessels
and remove the sensitiveness to changes of temperature after a warm bath. Then the douche, and
especially the "Scotch" douche with alternately
hot and cold water, being given with a tolerably
powerful stream has also, both by its thermic and
by its mechanical action, an effect on resorption
which, in many cases and especially in some joint-
affections, makes it a very valuable addition to the
massage treatment, the physiological effects of
which it to some extent participates.

In most well-regulated houses in Carlsbad tubs
are to be had for sitting baths, or for the cold,
morning sponge-bath. This latter bath, taken every
morning immediately after rising, forms an excellent habit, apt to keep up a healthy condition of
the skin and to preserve good nerves, and better
weak ones. But the temperature must suit the
individual, and it is a common mistake to think
that the colder the water the more beneficial are
its effects. The bath ought generally to be about
the temperature of the room. It must refresh
the patient as a cold bath but not be so cold as
to cause him to dread it or to give him a shock,

and for many an unaccustomed or a sensitive
person it may be advantageous to add some hot
water to the cold hygienic morning bath in order
to raise its temperature some few degrees above
that of the room. The cold morning bath ought
to last from one to two minutes.

The patients should carefully follow their physicians' prescriptions as to the frequency, the temperature, and the duration of their baths. This is
especially very necessary concerning mud-baths
and all hot baths—which, by the way, few people
ought to take oftener than every second day. All
the thermometers in the bath-houses, as elsewhere
in Carlsbad, are graduated after the Réaumur-sys-
tem, wherefore I have here used the figures of that
system. The best part of the day for bathing in
Carlsbad is from eleven o'clock A.M. until one
o'clock, P.M., and it will often be necessary to
secure a ticket early in the morning in order to get
a bath during that time. The patients must always
observe the universal rules not to bathe too soon
after a meal, or after strong bodily exercise, and
must themselves with the thermometer control the
temperature of the bath.

.   .   .   .   .   .

The *hills* around Carlsbad are of no small value
from a therapeutic point of view, and afford excellent opportunity for the of late very much used (and
very much misused), *s. c. Oertel terrain-cure*, for
which I refer the reader to what is said about
the cure for adiposity (p. 51). The wood-covered

heights form a most beautiful landscape, intersected in every direction by comfortable roads at every angle of declivity, and with numerous resting-places at short intervals.

.   . ～   .   .   .   .

In Carlsbad, as in the whole civilized world, the *mechanical treatment* of *gymnastics*, and above all, of *massage*, has been of late very much in vogue—and there can be no doubt that this treatment, much misused, falsely advertised, and badly represented as it has been and still is, forms a most important and effective part of therapeutics. It is in the nature of this treatment that it *must* to a certain extent be performed by persons without any medical knowledge, the medical profession not commanding the necessary number of hands for the mere mechanical work thus needed. But the public must be made aware of the fact that these "masseurs" and "masseuses," perfectly ignorant medically, are unable to make a diagnosis, unable to determine the indications for, or the possible dangers of, massage, unable to understand but in a very general way how it is to be performed, and above all unable to understand that they do not understand, and to appreciate the danger of their own ignorance. In fact, that mechanical quackery of persons without even the slightest medical education undertaking not only the mechanical part of mechano-therapy, but everything else belonging to it except knowledge and skill, has often at Carlsbad as elsewhere proved to be a very dangerous thing, and still oftener entirely misses its therapeutic purpose. Massage should, like every other treatment, never be performed but under the direction of a physician, and will in a great number of cases (in most cases of *s. c.* local massage) be effectively performed only by a physician. It is a pretty plain matter that only the person who performs it can be responsible for the manner in which it is performed—which I here point out not without my good reasons for doing so.

. . . . . .

The *physicians* in Carlsbad amounted, 1892, to the respectable number of sixty-nine. They all have that in common that they are Austrian subjects, and they all have acquired a diploma at some Austrian university. On account of the formerly often marked difficulty for the visitor-patient in Carlsbad of learning the address of any physician (except the physician of the house), every house in Carlsbad now has, or ought to have, on the premises, a printed list of all the physicians' names in alphabetical order, together with their addresses.

. . . . . .

I have saved for the last that therapeutic resource of Carlsbad which some people, not without good reasons, may consider its very first and best. I mean *the strong traditional discipline* in dietetics and hygiene pervading the place and exercising its moral influence on the patient ; and

3

I believe that Carlsbad has very few if any rivals in this respect outside of Austria. One would indeed meet with great, not to say with insurmountable, difficulties in bringing about anything similar in many other countries, and especially in those countries where an English or an American public regulates the style of life. In Carlsbad almost every consideration gives way to sanitary interests, and the whole community conforms to the interests of the "cure." Even now, when thirty-five thousand visitors, to a great part belonging to the upper classes, congregate there from all parts of the civilized world, the Bohemian village continues to wear much more the aspect of a resort for health than of one for fashion. Every one observes early hours, and the stranger follows the general example. In the restaurants the food is of excellent quality but simply prepared, and the bill of fare is based on dietetic principles, which are more or less known to every inhabitant of Carlsbad.[1] It is quite interesting to observe

[1] If these principles and other things belonging to medical science get mixed up during their circulation among the public with a good many superstitious ideas, this has practically no bad results. It is to me somewhat of a mystery that anybody in his senses can believe that, if he drinks Carlsbad-water in the morning or at any time, and afterwards swallows a cherry during the course of the day, the fruit will get impregnated with the carbonate of lime and remain as a concrement in the stomach,—but this queer idea prevents many people from eating raw fruits during their cure, which, *per se*, is a good thing. It is astounding to listen to some people's notions

how the sanitary interests and the hygienic discipline rule the place and exercise their influence
upon certain classes of patients, and how they
facilitate the physician's often difficult task.   The
young lady who devotes her whole interest and
sacrifices her health to social pleasures and
"duties" in some big western city, and who is
accustomed to rise at 11 A.M. and to go to bed at
2 A.M., in Carlsbad submits to a much healthier
system of living, comforting herself for the "awful
dulness" with the hope of eclipsing the next
winter every record of female loveliness.   The
two-hundred-and-fifty-pounder who is accustomed
to pass his time almost exclusively in bed, on
the sofa, or at the table, and to live on enormous
quantities of fattening things, contents himself
with an appropriate diet, and a puffing walk up
the hills of four hours a day.   The patient who
by his friends is mildly reproached for taking too
much stimulant, who by his enemies is declared
to be an habitual drinker, or even a drunkard, and
who generally declares himself that he is accustomed to take a drink when he feels he wants to
be "picked up" (and he may feel that want every
second hour), in Carlsbad becomes amenable to
treatment, and with trembling hands only carries
that quantity of alcoholic liquor to his lips which

about the danger of a nap in the afternoon during the cure,
but these wonderful fancies prevent many persons from sleep-
ing during the daytime, who ought to sleep only during the
night.

his physician thinks necessary to keep off any possible dangers of too sudden a change. And in this exceptionally strong moral influence on the patients lies a not inconsiderable part of the reasons of Carlsbad's unrivalled fame as a curing place, and of its often exceedingly beneficial influence on the patient, an influence which is well supported by the absence from the work and the exertions of home-life, by the freedom from social restraints, by the change of climate and of altitude, the living chiefly out-of-doors, and other like advantages, which Carlsbad shares with most other curing places.

THE DIET AND SOME OTHER MEDICAL TOPICS.

Most people who go to Carlsbad have a sanitary purpose for so doing, and every one who goes there for his health must fully understand that, if the "cure" is to have the wished-for result, some dietetic and other rules have to be observed, even if they impose some sacrifices upon the patient.

The diet is especially important, partly because it is a necessary item of the treatment in most "Carlsbad-diseases," partly because the use of the alkaline-saline water, *per se*, must be accompanied by a certain diet, the mucous membrane of the stomach getting much more sensitive under its influence that it generally is.

In trying to treat this matter at the same time as briefly as is necessary in a work of this kind and still in such a way that the reader may derive some use from the exposition, we immediately strike a difficulty in giving general rules for things, which must be more or less modified in every special case.

The best possible bill of fare for one diabetic patient may be very different from the best possible bill of fare for another patient of the same kind. The same fact is true of patients with ulcer of the stomach and of almost all the patients of different classes who visit Carlsbad. Still there are some rules which every one must observe. We will therefore first consider those, and then pass on to the rules for special diseases.

To begin from the beginning : no one ought to overcharge the stomach either by eating or drinking. It is therefore necessary that all the three meals of the day should be of some nutritive value ; that system which makes dinner the only real meal and reduces breakfast to a cup of coffee and a couple of biscuits and supper to something similar, is always a bad system (but rarely to be found in English or American people, I acknowledge). One must enjoy the pleasures of the table only until hunger and thirst are fully satisfied and no more. On the other hand I must remind the reader that the nonsensical starvation-system which prevailed some decades ago has only a historical interest, and has long since given place to more rational views, and to a fully satisfactory table.

Then we have some qualitative restrictions, which are good to remember. Some of them find (a rather inadequate and inexact) expression in the old saying : " Nothing sour, nothing salt, nothing sweet, nothing fat." This only means, practically, that we avoid some (not all) things, which possess any of those qualities in a very high degree. Then we also forbid all very hot or very cold things and all very spiced things. If we, moreover forbid too many starchy (or floury) things (*e. g.* puddings) and all raw fruits, we have with the greatest possible brevity said about all that can be said in such a general way concerning the solid foods.

The Americans expect a veto against ham—but do not get it. The ham in Carlsbad is very little salted and very little smoked and is an easily digested and a wholesome food. The calf also enjoys in Europe a better reputation for the meat it yields than it does in America. I am unable to ascribe a reason for this, if it be not that Americans often think the meat of the calf much more difficult of digestion than it really is.

As to liquids we forbid coffee entirely in a great many cases, generally without fearing very dangerous consequences if people commit a transgression now and then with " kafé verkehrt " (= coffee with a strong addition of milk), but keep our absolute veto against " kafé rechs " (= coffee with a small quantity of milk), and still more against " schwarzer kafé " (= black coffee). Coffee irritates, through its great quantity of empyreumatic substances, the mucous membrane of the stomach, and is a much less innocent beverage than most coffee-drinkers will believe ; taken in large quantities and concentrated it often causes catarrhs of the stomach and dyspepsia. Tea is in this respect much better, and contains the same stimulating alkaloid as coffee (which mankind discovered wherever it existed before the chemists had any idea of it). Thus we recommend tea for breakfast, not too strong but as weak

as you wish—still weaker in the evening and then
only for people whose sleep it does not disturb.
Chocolate or cocoa is in most cases permitted
(not in cases of diabetes or adiposity). The light
Pilsner beer is generally allowed in moderate quantities ; the light claret is rarely forbidden. The
strong wines, liquors, punches, cocktails, and kindred drinks, are forbidden ; brandy, gin, and
whiskey make a good Carlsbad-patient's hair stand
on end—especially if those liquors are not very
strongly diluted.

No Carlsbad-patient—or anybody else—ought to
smoke to excess ; those who are accustomed to
tobacco may indulge in one cigar after breakfast
and another after dinner. I take this occasion to
point out to heavy smokers that the cigar is a less
dangerous enemy to their health than the pipe or
—above all—than the cigarette. The cigarette-
smoker goes easily to excesses, controls with more
difficulty the quantity of tobacco consumed, and it
is a significant fact that among cigarette-smokers
there are oftener found the bad effects of
excessive use of tobacco, culminating in that sad
thing which the medical profession calls a " smoker's heart." The dyspeptic troubles that often attack hard smokers lead them to Carlsbad, which—
may it be said in parenthesis—is not a bad place
for wearing-off and overcoming the effects of excessive smoking.

In submitting to these rules the patients with
catarrh of the stomach or the bowels fulfil their

dietetic duties. The chronic interstitial inflammation of the kidney (and also the catarrh of the
bladder) makes it important for the patients to
avoid spices and to limit their beverage to milk,
chocolate, diluted claret, mineral waters, and
plain water and to abstain from all other drinks.
The hyperæmia of the liver and the fatty liver
generally impose the same duties as adiposity.
The rest of the " Carlsbad-diseases " deserve some
special words about the necessary dietetic rules.

. . . . . .

Ulcer of the Stomach (or of the Duodenum)

—is now, since the results of Leube's elaborate
researches were published, treated by a much better
diet than the former exclusive milk diet. This
modern diet promotes the healing process equally
well, and is far more apt to keep the patient in
good appetite and to maintain his bodily weight
and strength.

The details of the bill-of-fare for these patients
are chiefly determined by the time that has passed
since a hemorrhage has occurred (if it has occurred
at all), and by the existing symptoms and the con-
clusions we may draw from them concerning the
scar which the ulcer has left. If everything looks
well we successively enlarge the bill-of-fare ; if
any symptoms arise threatening a breaking up
of the scar and a new hemorrhage, we again
make restrictions. These patients generally appear in Carlsbad several weeks after a bleeding has
taken place, and it is then usually advisable to

allow them all the items of the following bill-of-fare, of which they during the first time after the hemorrhage could with safety only enjoy a very small part. When a month has passed after the hemorrhage, and the healing process seems to have been undisturbed, the patient's bill-of-fare comprises : Milk, tea, beef-tea or solution of beef, bouillon, English cakes, raw or softly boiled eggs, rice or sago well cooked in milk, mashed potatoes, brains, sweetbread, chickens, partridges, pigeons (boiled or broiled), raw ham or beef, calf's feet, venison, roast beef, beef-steak (or rump steak), lean fishes (not eel, herring, or salmon), macaroni, white bread, cooked fruits, wines (not the sweet kinds), and mineral waters.

[The above list may be relied upon for other therapeutic purposes than the healing of an ulcer in some cases where it is necessary to keep a strict diet—it only contains those foods which are easiest of digestion.]

The patients with ulcer of the stomach ought never to drink large quantities of water at a time, but ought to drink several times during the day. They ought to avoid violent exercises and physical efforts of all kinds. Their meals must always be moderate in quantity, and their dietetic duties are of paramount importance.

.   .   .   .   .   .

Patients with Dilatation of the Stomach must, when their disease is with certainty diagnosticated, prepare to follow a certain diet for the rest of their lives, and the resolution to do this ought to be so much the easier as they otherwise can never expect to see the symptoms of their dilatation disappear.

It is above all important for these patients never to take at a time any great amount of either liquid or solid food. It is not only a question of not "overcharging" the stomach in the ordinary sense of the expression, for even such quantities as are quite moderate and permissible for a normal stomach are too large for a dilated one. It is also necessary to take only such things as, in relation to their volume and their weight, have a high nutritive value. Whether the food is digested in the stomach or in the bowels, it stays longer than is normal in the former, and tends, if heavy, furthermore to dilate it.

The system, therefore, is as follows : many small meals of easily digested and very nutritious things every day. I generally prescribe one meal between breakfast and dinner, and one between dinner and supper,[1] and I recommend easily digested things varying according to the individual circumstances for each meal. For instance, at 9 A.M. a small cup of tea, one roll, a piece of meat or very often of raw beef, scraped or well hashed ; at 11:30 A.M. one egg, one half glass of milk or solution of meat (Maggis), a biscuit ; at 2 P.M.

[1] In Carlsbad we call breakfast the meal at about 9 A.M., dinner the meal at about 2 P.M., and supper the meal about 7:30 P.M.

half a chicken with some rice, a glass of claret, one half roll ; at 4:30 P.M. an egg with a biscuit and half a glass of milk ; at 7:30 P.M. a small piece of beef or fish, one roll, half a glass of milk. It is very often necessary to give the patient artificial means for facilitating the impaired digestion.

The Carlsbad-waters must be given in quite small but repeated quantities — say 120 c.c. one hour before breakfast, dinner, and supper.

But the stomach-dilatation patients can expect nothing more of the Carlsbad-waters than an in-crease of appetite and a decrease in their dyspeptic troubles and in the symptoms arising from the gastric catarrh ; it will not in the least affect the dilatation *per se.* For this we have other remedies, and the leisure at Carlsbad affords an excellent opportunity for the patient to learn how to wash out his stomach himself every morning immedi-ately after rising, and thus to rid it of the accumu-lated mucus and of remains of the food taken the day before. This is an extremely important item in the treatment of the dilatation of the stomach. The patient generally at first finds the whole pro-cedure rather unpleasant, but at the same time highly approves of the effect, and soon learns how to perform the washing, and gets used to it.

As another important remedy I must name the massage of the accessible part of the dilated stomach through the abdominal wall—it sometimes brings about a strong improvement in cases in which every other treatment has proved unsuccessful. For my part I have much less confidence in the faradisation of the stomach, but, as it is easy to perform, I have sometimes used it immediately before or after the massage.

.   .   .   .   .   .

The Gall-Stone-Patient is, under ordinary circumstances, scarcely any patient at all, which fact some physicians no less than patients would do well to remember. The causes of the formation of gall-stones are hitherto (except as far as me-chanical causes are concerned) very imperfectly known. The great probability that a catarrh of the gall-bladder or of the gall-ducts often has a part in their formation must not be forgotten in dietetic prescriptions, and makes it important for the patient to avoid things which may cause or main-tain a catarrh in the stomach, whence it may spread *per continuitatem* to the duodenum and to the gall-ducts. The gall-stone patient ought thus to follow those general dietetic rules which are common to all Carlsbad-patients, and which in fact everybody, in or outside Carlsbad, would do well to observe. But under ordinary circumstances this is enough. As long as the gall flows freely, the mere existence of a gall-stone in the gall-bladder does not prevent digestion from being perfectly physiological (even as to the resorption of fat) ; such a patient (who may live through a long life without ever having any trouble from his gall-stones) ought to be put under no *special* restric-tions. I take the liberty of pointing this out especially because I have repeatedly seen gall-stone patients put on such a "strict" diet that they have by this and by this alone lost enormously in flesh and in general health, and fallen into a neurasthenic state, which, *per se*, has been a much greater burden than many gall-stones are to their respective bearers.

When the flow of gall is prevented by the passage or by the impaction of a gall-stone, then is the time for dietetic restrictions. They are then indicated sometimes by the sensitiveness of the stomach, which on these occasions only stands the easiest digested things in small quantities, and often by the want of gall in the bowel, and the consequent imperfect resorption of fat, for which reason fat ought then to be avoided.

The gall-stone patient is often cured in Carlsbad. But it is just as unjustifiable to promise him a certain and complete cure as it is to tell him that he *must* under all circumstances come to Carlsbad three consecutive years. He may be cured in one year, and he may not be cured in many years.

.   .   .   .   .   .

Adiposity is treated in different ways by different physicians, but the systems are so far alike that they all recur to means of two kinds : (1) a certain diet ; and (2) locomotion.

In these cases again the physician meets with the ever recurring necessity of not struggling so hard in one direction and for one purpose as to forget other very important interests. By too

rapid and too great a loss of fat we incur certain
dangers of disturbing the heart, the .nervous
system, and the general health and strength—and
for every adipose patient there exists a (varying)ʻ
limit both as to the rate and as to the quantity of
the loss of weight, which he cannot exceed without serious, sometimes very serious, consequences.
The individual differences in this respect are very
great and it is impossible to give any figures of a
general value.   I have seen a decrease of one
pound a day on the average for five weeks without
any other than healthy consequences.   But in
most cases I would be unwilling to take more than
about twelve per cent. of a patient's weight during a
" cure " at Carlsbad, and unwilling to cause such a
loss in less time than two months.¹   In a great
many cases where weak nerves, weak hearts, and
an indifferent state of general health are concerned,
the cure must be slower and the reduction smaller.

The diet ought to represent such a restriction in
the amount of those kinds of food which chiefly
contribute to the formation of fat, that the
organism, mostly on account of increased locomotion, is forced to recur for its support to the fat
already formed.   In all the different cure-systems

¹ During a longer time a much greater loss of weight may
sometimes be brought about.   When this goes to the press I
meet a former patient, a short lady, who in 1891, during and
after a Carlsbad cure, decreased from 211 to 151 pounds.
Since then she keeps the latter weight, and is very much
improved in general health.

(Harvey, Voit, Ebstein, Demuth, Oertel, Schven-
ninger) we find in different degrees a restriction of
fat, or of carbo-hydrates (sugar and starch), or of
both these classes of food.

To bring about a reasonable and not too quick
or too great a loss of flesh, I, for my part, generally
forbid all the fattest kinds of food—all fat, butter,
cream, cheese, and milk, pork and ham, goose and
duck, rich sauces, salmon, eel, herring, lobster, and
crabs. In point of starch and sugar, all pure sugar
and all sweets are forbidden, likewise puddings,
cakes, potatoes, peas, beans, rice, macaroni, corn,
sago, tapioca, arrow-root, etc. Then, and above all,
it is necessary to *fix* the daily portion of bread for
the patient, who should never be allowed more than
a very moderate quantity daily.

So much about the solid food. I now arrive at
a most important question about the rational treatment of adipose patients—a question that has of
late been pushed to the front, and about the importance of which it has become an urgent necessity as far as possible to enlighten the public. During the last few decades the reduction of the daily
quantity of drinking-water has been tried by some
German physicians in the treatment of adiposity
and has been widely adopted by the public. A
great many fat people now follow out this part of
the treatment, sometimes even without consulting
any physician—either by avoiding all drinking at
meals, or by restricting the whole daily quantity of
drinking-water, or by observing both these rules.

I cannot in a work of this nature at length expatiate on all the many evil results which in most cases must be the consequences of this violence to nature. By not drinking at meals one easily causes loss of appetite and dyspeptic troubles ; the very fact that this restriction very quickly causes a loss of flesh shows that the universal custom of all mankind to dilute the gastric juice and the contents of the stomach at meals by water is not an accidental thing but has its good reasons and is beneficial to the digestion and assimilation. As for the restriction of the whole daily quantity beyond a very fair allowance, it cannot be effected without great disturbance in many physical and chemical processes in the organism. It is an especially favorable method for bringing about a gouty condition, by not permitting the satisfactory elimination of useless and obnoxious products of the metamorphosis of substances ; by concentrating secretions and excretions it may cause the formation of concrements in the gall or in the urine ; carried to an extreme degree it must inevitably diminish the whole mass of blood, lower the intra-arterial pressure, and unfavorably change the conditions for the functions of the heart, while experience often shows it to have a most disastrous influence upon the whole nervous system,—finally, it is proved that this unfortunate method, probably owing to the changed and concentrated state of the urine, in a great percentage of cases may bring on an inflammation of the kidneys.

4

In denouncing this greatly abused restriction of water as far as it is used against adiposity *per se* and in cases where the heart is still able to fulfil its functions [1] I must add that it is further-more entirely superfluous in every case where the patient has the full use of his lower limbs. In these cases we can always, by other dietetic means and by locomotion, bring about the full loss of fat which the patient can bear without injury to his health. I therefore entirely condemn this sys-tem, and sincerely hope that we will soon see the last of it. I advise the great majority of my own patients to regulate the daily quantity of water according to their thirst, and especially to drink at meals.

On the other hand, the adipose patient ought to drink as little alcoholic liquors as possible, and I generally restrict those to a quantity which a con-tinued habit to drink them may have made neces-sary.

The other important item in the treatment for adiposity is, as I have already said, locomotion—either by a systematic exercise of the organs of locomotion, *i. e.*, by gymnastics, or by walking.

---

[1] In certain cases of heart diseases in which the heart has lost the full power of fulfilling its functions, a moderate re-striction in the daily quantity of drinking-water may be ad-vised. This restriction can never be carried to an extreme point on account of the beforementioned serious reasons ; its indication and its reasonable extent can only be determined by an experienced physician.

During the last years there has been made a very extensive therapeutic use of the mechanical task that climbing imposes upon the organism, partly as an item in the cure of adiposity and partly as an important part in the treatment of some diseases of the heart. And this leads us to the contemplation of a very satisfactory feature in modern mechano-therapy, which is known as the

Terrain-Cure,

and which in Carlsbad rationally represents the locomotive part of the adipose patient's therapeutic duties. The cure consists in daily walking a certain distance over the hills, which increases the muscular task, strengthens the muscles, and contributes to the consumption of fat more than the walking on even ground. It makes respiration deeper, and has an important influence on the heart, which we will, with a few passing words, take into consideration. The heart is, as we all know, a muscle, which has for its function the keeping up of the circulation by driving the blood through the vessels. By climbing we increase the work of the heart and by systematically giving it this increased task we influence it in the same way that we influence a muscle by exercising it—*i. e.*, we transfer to it through its own arteries a larger amount of blood, heighten its state of nutrition, increase its volume, and strengthen it generally. Thus climbing has been recommended to persons with weak hearts and to persons with organic heart-diseases in certain

stages. This is one side of the medal, and a pleasant one to contemplate. On the other side, we
must notice that the heart may, as well as any other
muscle, become overstrained—and there is not the
slightest doubt that some people have, in the first
throb of delight over the *s. c.* " Oertel terrain-
cure " committed frightful errors by straining
weak hearts and by giving them too hard a func-
tional task, thus dilating and weakening instead of
strengthening them. Then there are certain affec-
tions· of the heart and vessels, which, form very
serious contra-indications against every terrain-
cure.

The cure seems to be the simplest thing in the
world—especially if we overlook some unnecessary
and some quite nonsensical little decorations
wherewith it has lately been garnished. Still it is
anything but simple, and belongs most decidedly to
those things the patient should never undertake
on his own risk or without the superintendence of
a physician. On the other hand, nobody can understand as well as the patient if his heart for the
moment is overstrained by his climbing or not.
He must only know that, as soon as he gets very
short of breath, his heart has a difficult task, and
he must then stop to take rest until he feels his
respiration in good order again. Thus these patients ought successively to increase the length of
their daily walks in the hills, to climb more and
more, to perform for every week an increased mechanical work—but to climb slowly and to rest

often. There are splendid opportunities in Carlsbad for the terrain-cure—the place being surrounded by endless walks in charming surroundings, where much has been done for the visitor's comfort, pleasure, and perfect personal safety.

.   .   .   .   .   .

The Gouty Patient has some duties, which in different countries and by different physicians are somewhat differently estimated. In spite of this difference of opinions there are certain points about which all must agree.

The gouty patient must, above all, very moderately enjoy the pleasures of the table and live on what is commonly called plain food, and finds in this general rule his most important prescriptions. On the bill-of-fare, the meat and in general albuminous food must be represented in moderate quantities ; fat things (especially cheese) ought also to be sparingly indulged in ; cooked fruits and green vegetables should have a prominent place. In some places one has (after Cantani) gone still further and urged a restriction also in the carbohydrates. This latter view we only adopt as far as sugar is concerned, the rigid restriction of which seems rational for several reasons and especially on account of the affinity, which there certainly exists between gout and diabetes, and the *rôle* that too much eating of sweets is considered to play in the etiology of this last disease.

Strongly spiced things ought to be avoided ; coffee and tea moderately partaken of ; alcoholic liquors are sometimes entirely forbidden—when long custom has made them necessary only a moderate quantity must be allowed and even that quantity only in a very diluted form.

The sacrifices which the patient must submit to must follow the lines indicated above. But too many restrictions are dangerous ; and those that are imposed must be based upon the individual circumstances, and with due consideration for the patient's customs, especially if these patients are advanced in life and have for many years had rather luxurious dietetic habits. It will not do to impose too poor a table in such cases, for the patient then risks losing much more in appetite, health, and general strength than he gains from the diminishing of the gouty diathesis, and risks changing this latter affection into severer forms.—The gouty patient ought to have much locomotion and to drink much water.

.   .   .   .

The Cure for Diabetes consists in a very great part in a certain dietetic *régime*, which is always exceedingly important to the patient—even if it ought not, as exclusively as many patients (and some physicians) think, make up the *whole* treatment.

In the dietetic treatment of diabetes, two faults are common. The one, and less common, fault is to follow a too strict diet of exclusively animal food. I cannot in a work of this nature elaborately present the possible dangers of the so-called absolute diabetic diet,[1] or lecture on the few and passing indications for such a diet, which may arise. I must restrict myself to say that in the great majority of cases there is reason for permitting the patient some vegetables and some bread.

Another fault in the treatment of diabetes is to be entirely too free with the allowance of carbohydrates [2]—this fault is a much commoner one than

[1] For my part I am averse to the exclusively animal diet, especially in those severer forms of the disease, in which such a diet does not make the sugar disappear, but where it always increases other substances in the blood (and urine) which are more injurious than the glucose and materially increase the danger of the state we call "coma diabeticum." In the lighter forms of diabetes there may arise passing indications for an absolute animal diet, as when one wishes suddenly to reduce an excessive amount of glucose, or when the patient passes through some healing process, or in the very beginning of a diabetes or a glucosuria, when such a diet may even bring about a recovery. But just as certain as it is that the strength and general health improve in a patient, who passes from a too free to a more strict diet, just so certain it is that the reverse takes place, if this same patient, (especially if the glucose is formed in him from albuminous substances), is put on an exclusively animal diet.

[2] The carbo-hydrates which belong to the human food consist of the different kinds of sugar and of starch, which in all (even healthy) people, chiefly through the influence of the pancreatic juice, form glucose in the digestive apparatus and which in diabetic people more or less exclusively pass through the blood and appear in the urine as glucose. The hydro-

the former. By too free an allowance of carbo-hydrates the glucose in the blood is unnecessarily increased, the patient falls into a state of diminished power of resistance to some dangers which constantly threaten him, and besides promotes the development from a milder into a severer form of his disease.

Every physician, who has given his careful attention to diabetes and who has had a large material at his disposition, will accede to the old general rule : the diabetic patient must chiefly live on albuminous substances and on fat, and must conform to some restrictions in the third great class of foods—carbo-hydrates (= sugar and starch),—a rule which may also be expressed thus : the diabetic patient must diet chiefly on animals and only to a very small degree on plants. The older the patient and the milder the form of his disease, the smaller, as a rule, are the privations he must be subjected to. Thus we find also in these cases the necessity to individualize, and that each case has, so to speak, its own rational bill-of-fare. Still the dietetic prescriptions can to a certain extent be generalized.

Every diabetic patient may, without any special restrictions, eat any otherwise healthy animal food *except* milk and liver. He is thus welcome to meats,

carbons belong chiefly to plants. In animals, milk contains about 5 per cent. of milk-sugar, or lactose, and the liver contains some (varying) per cents. of glycogen, which has been called animal starch. All kinds of flour largely contain starch.

birds, and fishes of all kinds, eggs, oysters,[1] crabs, scallops, lobsters, clams, turtle, terrapin, and caviare. · He ought to be liberal with himself in regard to fat substances, cheese, butter ; one glass of rich cream [2] a day may also be allowed.

Of the articles of food derived from plants we may, from a practical point of view, distinguish several groups. Every wise diabetic patient will forever bid farewell to certain things which, without giving him any advantages or being in any way necessary to his well-being, strongly increase the amount of glucose. He will thus abstain from all kinds of sweets, from sugar and syrup and everything that contains any considerable amount of such a substance, from rice, indian corn, arrowroot, sago, tapioca, from all puddings and all things made of or strongly mixed with flour ("macaroni," "nudeln," etc.), from peas, beans, turnips, artichokes, sweet potatoes, chestnuts, carrots, parsnips, beets, bananas, pineapples, figs, dates, grapes, and also in general from all *dried* fruits *except* almonds and nuts (see below — *i.e.* wal-

---

[1] Oysters and other "shell-fish" have a liver, and in eating them the diabetic patient gets a small amount of glycogen. But the amount is *so* small that I do not consider it wise to deprive a patient of these refreshing dishes, who in other respects must be put under so many restrictions.

[2] The milk contains, as already stated, about ˙5 per cent. of milk-sugar. But rich cream contains less sugar but much easily digested, fat ; and a large glass of cream every morning at breakfast goes far to keep the thin diabetic patient from growing thinner—if cream otherwise agrees with him.

nuts, para- and cocoa-nuts, hazel-nuts, etc.). Potatoes are often enumerated as entirely objectionable, yet many persons are so accustomed to them that they feel great difficulty in entirely forsaking them. The cooked potato contains about 15½ per cent. of starch—a pretty large percentage, but only about half as much as peas and beans and only about one fifth of what rice contains. I am therefore willing in light (but only in light) cases of diabetes, to permit the patient a very moderate (and in quantity fully determined) use of potatoes.

In greater or smaller quantity, according to the age of the patient, the state of the disease and other circumstances, one may also now and then permit many a diabetic patient some amount of sour apples (rather than pears), of oranges, grapefruits, lemons, peaches, apricots, plums, sour cherries, the different kinds of berries (cranberries, raspberries, strawberries, blueberries, etc.), muskmelons, watermelons, squashes, pumpkins, cucumbers, the whole (very eatable) pods of peas, string-beans, the leaves of the different kinds of cabbages, horse-radishes, radishes, eggplants, oysterplants, tomatoes, olives, asparagus, salad, spinach, celery, chicory (leaves), watercresses and other green vegetables, mushrooms, almonds, and nuts. This list ought to make an exceedingly satisfactory impression on every diabetic—but ought to be read with a special attention to the introductory lines of this little piece, which form a most important part of it.

The bread takes a peculiar position and deserves to be especially mentioned at some greater length. It chiefly consists of starch and can never be permitted in any large or unlimited quantity. But the human stomach is so used to it that the complete abstinence from it is a very severe privation, and besides often causes serious troubles of the stomach and bowels. We must therefore make a compromise between the different needs which make themselves felt in this matter and—except in those few cases in which an absolute animal diet may for some time seem rational—allow a certain quantity of bread. It is very important that this quantity be well fixed, and I therefore am accustomed to order it to be weighed out for the patient every morning, and to forbid all supplies from other quarters.

Many endeavors have been made to produce a bread for diabetic patients, which should at the same time give them a very small amount of starch and be a substitute as to taste for ordinary bread. This problem is yet to a certain extent as impossible of solution as the squaring of the circle. All of these many breads suffer from either one of two defects. Either they do not taste like real bread, or else they give the patient a large quantity of starch. The *real* gluten-bread is tasteless and, like the better inulin-bread, very dear. The graham-bread is excellent to taste but contains a very large amount of starch. This is also the case with a great many breads which often are given out to be free or nearly free from starch. The soya-bread contains above 23 per cent. of carbo-hydrates ; soya-biscuits, about twice as much ; some breads which are falsely called gluten-bread contain 49 per cent., others 55 per cent. thereof, the much-proclaimed "florador" 75½ per. cent., "semolina" 74½ per cent., the new "aleuronate"-bread contains over 66 per cent. of carbo-hydrates. By the sale of these breads, the real percentage of which is rarely mentioned, but which very often are given out as containing 2 to 3 per cent. of starch or something like it, diabetic people have been very badly served—the more so as they are always prone to persuade themselves that they may eat any amount of these kinds of bread. I think it high time for specialist-physicians to disclose the unscrupulous humbug who is financially benefited by these breads—to the great detriment of the diabetic patients.

For my part, I give my patients a certain amount of ordinary bread or a somewhat larger amount of graham bread. Sometimes I fill up the wished-for amount of bread by Seegen's [1] or Pavy's almond bread. These "breads" do not contain starch or

[1] The powder of one quarter pound dried and finely pulverized almonds is put in a linen bag and cooked a quarter of an hour in water with some drops of vinegar, then well kneaded with three and a half ounces of butter and two whole eggs. Then the yolks of three other eggs and some salt are added to the mass. The three whites of the eggs are well beaten and also added, whereupon the whole is put in some buttered form and baked.

any considerable quantity of sugar, and taste tolerably good ; their defects are that they are not
easily digested and are very dear. Together with real
bread they may often make a good supply and be
a not unpleasant substratum for butter and cheese.

Of the fluids we entirely forbid porter, beer,[1] and
ale of all kinds and, above all, champagne ("sweet"
and " dry"), also strong and sweet wines (port,
madeira, malaga, sherry, marsala, malvasia, tokay,
muscatel, angelica, constantia, etc.), then punch,
fruit-wines, and "liqueurs" of all kinds, together
with chocolate. Light red and white wines are
permitted (claret rather than burgundy, all the
Rhine wines, but not sauterne, graves or barsac).
Of American wines, the Virginia claret, the catawba
wines, and many California wines (riesling, zin-
fandel, burgundy, etc.) contain only small quantities
of glucose, and may be used. Brandy, whiskey, and
kindred drinks are permitted to the diabetic patient
—but, of course, only in very moderate quantities,
and only diluted by water.

The last few years have produced for diabetics
a substitute, as far as taste is concerned, for sugar,
in the well known saccharine, which is sold in most
drug stores in small tablets, of which one is enough

---

[1] I forbid all my diabetic people beer, even the light
Pilsner. It gives comparatively much glucose. If the
patients drink it at all they are inclined to drink large quantities of it, and it is not necessary to anybody's well-being.
A thin brandy or whiskey (soda-water) grog serves the diabetic's purpose much better.

to sweeten a cup of tea or of coffee. Saccharine has been accused of having some bad qualities and effects, but these accusations seem to me to remain—as far as small quantities are concerned—unproved, and may, perhaps, be a result brought about by certain interested individuals, who consider themselves threatened by this new cheap substitute for sugar. " Diabetine," another substitute for sugar, has just now made its appearance. I have not yet had time to form any opinion of it.

Diabetic persons should be specially careful to be frugal in everything which has an influence on the nervous system. Tea, coffee, and alcoholic liquors must be used in very small quantities. Smoking should be avoided, or reduced to a minimum. In my opinion, excesses in this direction sometimes play a *rôle* in the origin of the disease, and they certainly exercise a still more pernicious influence upon diabetic than upon other people.

It is very important for diabetic persons to avoid strains, excesses, and emotions of all kinds, and to arrange their lives as free from such influences and as easy as circumstances permit. Then the diabetic patient must give a special attention to avoid colds, and ought always to use flannel underwear. The other items in the treatment I must omit to mention in this place. But I will, for the sake of honesty and in the patient's own interest, state that the really diabetic patient can very rarely hope to be completely *cured* from his disease, and a promise to effect such a cure, either by the Carlsbad water or by any means whatever, is at this present day entirely unjustified and ought to awaken the patient's distrust. The diabetic patient in Carlsbad often increases his defective powers of assimilating carbo-hydrates, his thirst diminishes, the unpleasant dryness of his mouth disappears, he feels less nervous and more vigorous, etc., and he generally is himself satisfied with the result of the cure, *if* he has not come to the place with the erroneous idea that it will entirely relieve him of his disease, which, when it appears in a light form and in an advanced time of life is not necessarily likely to shorten or to darken life, and often more deserves to be called a weakness than a disease.

BEFORE AND AFTER THE CURE—THE NECESSARY TIME FOR A CARLSBAD-CURE.

People have talked and written a good deal about the "before-cure," the "Carlsbad-cure," and the "after-cure." It seems to me that this has happened more on account of the common human wish for division, and on account of the inexplicable (but existing) love for the number three, than on account of the facts as they really are.

"Before-cure" means nothing but the patient's submission to the dietetic rules of his case during some time before his arrival in Carlsbad. This submission is highly to be approved of, whether the patient goes to Carlsbad or not. His non-submission to the above-named rules does not prevent his going to Carlsbad and beginning the cure (and the submission) at once. I therefore think the word "before-cure" to be somewhat unnecessary. On the other hand, some people who intend to go to Carlsbad "make up" beforehand for the sacrifices they will have to make, thereby indulging more freely than ever in their darling dietetic sins—whether these are brought about by solid or by liquid temptations. If the word "before-cure" can bring those patients to a better understanding of their duties toward themselves before coming to Carlsbad, the word is useful enough to warrant its existence.

One need not be very intelligent to understand that a chronic disease of long standing must, of necessity, require a long use of healing remedies, whether in form of Carlsbad-waters, of dietetic or other hygienic rules, or in any other form. But a great many people who come to Carlsbad, and who are very intelligent in other matters, are rather dull, not to use a stronger expression, in this. The usual minimum of a Carlsbad cure is four weeks.[1] A great many patients stay a much longer time than this, which would, indeed, in most cases, be much too short if sanitary interests alone should prevail. It hardly ever enters into the head of a German, Scandinavian, or any other Continental visitor at Carlsbad, to come there with the purpose of staying less time than four weeks. But the English, and especially the Americans, very often wish to curtail even this minimum of four weeks, and it is not rare to hear them explain at the very beginning of their first interview with their physician that they can only give three weeks to the cure, which they somehow consider to be "about the ordinary time

---

[1] It is easy to prove that these four weeks are traditional as a minimum. When a visitor comes to Carlsbad and takes lodgings without any special agreement, the law expects that he has taken them for four weeks, obviously because visitors in Carlsbad hardly ever stay a shorter time than this.

5

for it." Let me say frankly that this is, in the great majority of cases, perfectly absurd. The visitor who comes to Carlsbad with any imperfection of his health at all, and with a sanitary purpose, ought to prepare for a longer stay there, and in scarcely any cases can a reasonable minimum of time be set at anything below four weeks.

The term **after-cure** has a better *raison d'être* than the term before-cure. The mucous membrane of the stomach gets much more sensitive under the influence of the alkaline-saline water than it usually is, and it retains that sensitiveness for some time. On account of this circumstance alone, it is reasonable to be somewhat more particular in dietetic matters just after a cure at Carlsbad than at other times, and to avoid raw fruits, very sour, or fat, or sweet, or salt, or smoked things (and I always add to my patients to avoid coffee) for some weeks. Then there are many patients who would do well to pass, between their stay at Carlsbad and their return to the duties, cares, and work of home, some weeks at an alpine or a sea-side or some other resort.

Carlsbad is open to visitors the year round. But the winter is a dreary time there, and only a very small percentage of the visitors are seen during the interval between the beginning of October and the end of April. The official season opens the first of May and closes the last of September. During the first part of May the temperature may be very chilly and people who go there then would do well to pre-

pare for this. The height of the season is from the
middle of June to the beginning of August. During
the latter part of August the season drops tolerably suddenly and in advanced September Carlsbad
is relatively empty.

Life in Carlsbad.

A visitor-patient in Carlsbad generally spends his
day in the following manner : He rarely rises later
than seven and he is generally at that time ready to
walk to his spring. He will there find a great many
other guests from different parts of the world and
will often, especially during the height of the season
be obliged to walk some time in procession, before
he, in his turn, gets his glass filled by some of the
little girls whom the town employs for this purpose.
After having drunk his prescribed number of glasses
—with at least fifteen minutes' interval after each
glass,—the patient walks leisurely around for about
an hour and then is ready for his breakfast, which
very often is taken somewhere out-of-doors at some
of the many restaurants, but which always can be
had at home, whether this is at a private house or
at a hotel. The typical Carlsbad-breakfast consists
of two soft-boiled eggs, two rolls and butter, some
cold ham, and a cup of tea or a glass of milk. The
time between breakfast and what is called dinner at
Carlsbad (but lunch by most English-speaking visitors) is mostly spent in walking, reading, cor-
responding, etc. The bathing patients ought to take

their bath before their dinner ; the afternoon and evening are, on account of the frequent and sudden changes of temperature, much less appropriate times for bathing. Those who are to take the "terrain-cure" ought to fulfil their duty in that respect before dinner, and those who want some rest or sleep during the course of the day should also do this before, rather than after this meal.

Dinner is rarely taken later than two o'clock P.M. It generally consists of some soup or fish, a sub-stantial portion of meat with vegetables, and of a compôt of cooked fruits. Many visitors drink the usual light Pilsner-beer, others the Austrian claret[1] —which is somewhat heavy and can bear some dilu-tion with Giesshübler or some other water.

The afternoon is chiefly devoted to leisure and pleasure. A part of the public enjoys the excellent musical performances which are always given in one place or another ; others make pedestrian or carriage trips to remarkable places in the neighborhood. The supper is taken at seven o'clock or a little later, and generally consists of some warm dish, or a couple of eggs with some bread and butter and cold meat, a glass of milk or a cup of tea or a glass of Pilsner-

---

[1] The Vöslauer, red or white, is the commonest of Austrian wines in Carlsbad, served in " pfiffs " at a low price and of ˎ modest quality, and in quart or pint bottles, which are of bet-ter quality. Vöslauer Goldeck is the ordinary better wine. Vöslauer Cabinet "grüne or blaugraue Etiquette " is the best, and is really quite a good wine. Besides these there are many others, Austrian or Hungarian, white and red wines.

beer [for which latter beverage the German visitor shows a decided preference]. After the supper, which is very often taken where the evening orchestra is playing (at Pupps' establishment, at the Stadtpark, at Goldener Schild, etc.,) there may still be time for a short walk. At nine o'clock P.M. the lively crowds suddenly begin to disappear, this being the legitimate time for retiring at Carlsbad—and at ten o'clock P.M. the streets are empty and quiet.

People go to Carlsbad chiefly for sanitary purposes, which, as already stated, are paramount to everything else in the place and entirely determine its character. The life at the great Bohemian health resort is more or less free and easy ; and the many partly absurd and often wearisome social gatherings and observations which sometimes prevail in places where a great many persons of means and position meet, entirely disappear at Carlsbad. The public pleasures (except excellent daily musical entertainments) are few and chiefly limited to the dramatical or lyrical performances at the theatre and the " reunions dansantes " (alias " hops ") at the Kurhaus every Saturday evening. Any person accustomed to a life of varied and elaborate diversions will find the day chiefly divided between sanitary exercises, walks, and meals somewhat monotonous. But the great majority of visitors soon get accustomed to, and afterwards have an endearing remembrance of, the simple, but healthy and, upon the whole, very pleasant life at Carlsbad.

The City of Carlsbad

is a small town of about 13,000 inhabitants located in the bottom and on the slopes of a little valley in the northwest corner of German Bohemia (which belongs to Austria), at 50° 13′ 11″ north latitude, and 12° 53′ 19″ east longitude ; 1,227 English feet above the sea, with 7.39° C. (= 45.3 Fahr.) average temperature of the year and 14° C. (= 57.2° Fahr.) average temperature of the time from the 1st of May until the 1st of October (= the " season"). The old parts of the town are built along the shores of the little river Tepl in the bottom of the valley, and we find there many old-fashioned houses and narrow streets ; in the outskirts of the town and higher úp on the slopes we generally find modern houses and broader streets.

Carlsbad is, during the season, to be reached in nine and a half hours from Berlin, five from Dresden, twenty-one from Bremen, ten and a quarter from Frankfurt-on-Main, eighteen and a half from Hamburg, seventeen and a quarter from Cologne, eleven from Vienna, thirty from Trieste, and twenty-nine from Paris.

If at this present moment there remain something for man to do for Carlsbad [1] from a hygienic point

---

[1] The imperfect canalization of the Tepl and the sewerage, which has left much to desire, have, among the many great improvements of the last decennium in Carlsbad, been rather weak points in the town. It is therefore with great satisfaction that we learn that a new and perfect system of sewerage has

of view, nature has provided it with great advantages, and it is upon the whole a very salubrious place. I cannot in truth confirm the familiar statement that epidemics never occur at Carlsbad. But only those infections which in every town are more or less common occur also in Carlsbad ; epidemics are rare ; there is no malaria, and there has hitherto been no cholera even when this plague has made ravages in Bohemia and in the immediate neighborhood of Carlsbad.

The surrounding hills reach very nearly 2,000 feet above the sea and are almost all thickly wooded up to the peaks. The vegetation is that common to middle Germany, and the trees are chiefly pines and firs, beeches, birches, and oaks. On account of the rich vegetation, the mountains, the distant views, the surroundings of Carlsbad are so beautiful that the visitor almost pardons the landscape its lack of all considerable bodies of water. No lakes are to be seen and the only rivers are the Eger and the insignificant little Tepl.

The inhabitants of the town amount, as already stated, to about 13,000, of which the great majority are Germans, only some few " Czechs," but more than 2,000 Hebrews. The plurality belongs to the Catholic religion, the rest (except the Jews) to the Protestant evangelic church. The whole population speaks German—a fact which is scarcely worth

been adopted by the authorities and is now under construction, so that the town will in this respect henceforth be perfectly well provided.

mentioning in this book on account of the wonderful capability of the Anglo-American for avoiding the mastering of any foreign language.

The character of the inhabitants of Carlsbad has been so much and so exclusively praised by some authors that I am somewhat at a loss here for a suitable manner of approaching this subject. Some philosophers say that man is morally the result of inherited qualities and of external circumstances. The inherited qualities of the Carlsbadians are those of the Germans in general, whom I consider to be a good people. They possess in a high degree that pleasant quality which they themselves call "Gemüthlichkeit," they are obedient to the laws, industrious, and (sometimes rather excessively) economical, they are as moral as some nations and very much less immoral than some other nations ; in short, I consider the inherited qualities of the Carlsbadians to be simply excellent. On the other hand, it has sometimes occurred to me that the population at watering places may not live under the most advantageous external circumstances for developing *all* the higher qualities of mankind. Just and equitable people, who like to see things as they are, should therefore not get exasperated with me if I state that I sometimes have found the inhabitants of Carlsbad not absolutely free from those little faults that usually prevent us from admiring too much the population of similar places.

One of the many good things in Carlsbad is this, that every relation between the population and the visitor is well regulated by law, which is cheaply and comfortably and very impartially and justly dealt out.[1] The visitor must remember the necessity of settling those points about which a dispute may arise, distinctly and completely beforehand, so that any agreement may be perfectly understood on both sides.

Carlsbad is a village in winter, but partakes of some of the qualities of a city in summer. The great majority of foreign visitors frequent the place between May 1st and the end of September, and during this period chiefly from the end of May to the end of August. The number of visitors has slowly increased so that it now amounts to about 35,000 a year. Of these there are over 2,000 Americans and over 1,000 Englishmen. The majority of visitors are Germans (from Austria or from Germany), and they give the crowd at the springs in the morning its general character. But representatives of every civilized (and some rather uncivilized) nations are found in Carlsbad, and the public somewhat alters its appearance according to the different national elements of which it is made up. In the spring we find a great quantity of Austrians, Germans, and

---

[1] Since I came to Austria I have three times been a witness before the law in controversies between natives and foreigners. All the three times it was a matter of unjust attack on the foreigner's purse by the natives, all the three times the court proposed a compromise, which every time was refused, and all the three times the case was justly and speedily decided in favor of the foreigner.

Scandinavians—the Russians are also early. During the height of the season—from the middle of June and into advanced August—Americans and English people are heard and seen all over the place. At the same time there are a good many slavonic-speaking visitors, and hundreds of the orthodox Polish Jews in their long coats and with their long curled hairlocks at the temples. A not inconsiderable number of visitors hail from the southeast part of Europe, and the sight of a red fez is not rare—now and then a full Oriental costume may be observed. Just after the middle of August the number of visitors suddenly decreases, and in October Carlsbad is almost deserted by foreign visitors.

Historic Notes.

Carlsbad is a very old town, belonged with the surrounding country to the Czechs and was called Vary. During the first part of the German time, which occurred at least as early as in the 13th century, it exchanged this name for its German translation, Warmbad. During the 14th century, in the reign of the Emperor Charles IV., the town got its present name.

People have spent a great deal of time and of trouble in ascertaining if the monarch (in hunting) discovered the springs, or if this glory should be denied him, and have thus come to the conclusion—which ought *a priori* to have been pretty clear to them—that the springs were known long before Charles IV. Yet he gave the city of Carlsbad (the 14th Aug., 1370) certain privileges, which the son Wenzel renewed and enlarged. The son Sigismund pawned the town to a Count Schlick, who seems, however, to have been obliged to conquer it for himself at some cost of blood and money. The Count also got out of pocket and sold the town to a Knight Polacky ; it returned only as late as 1547 to the Bohemian crown. The trials of the town were, however, not yet ended ; it has since been pawned a couple of times, and political and natural powers have disturbed its otherwise calm existence. At the time of the Reformation the Carlsbadians quickly and lustily adopted the reformed religion, but when the Emperor Ferdinand II., after the battle on the "White Mountain" (1620), made up his accounts with the Protestants, they (the Carlsbadians), with admirable presence of mind, made haste to become good Catholics again. This confessional plasticity may not have been to the taste of (my own dear ancestors) the Swedes, who were of sterner moods, and who made several rather long visits in Bohemia during the Thirty Years' War, sacked Carlsbad in 1640 and left here, as elsewhere in Bohemia, a frightful memory behind them. Since this time French and Prussian armies have left their cards at Carlsbad, the Prussians as late as 1866. The elements too have helped to disturb now and then the monotony of village life in Carlsbad. In the year 1604 the whole town (with the exception of three houses) was burnt; in the year 1759 luck was almost as bad, and our own century has also seen some big fires. The blessed springs have also now and then played some practical jokes on the Carlsbadians by the breaking out of its usual boundaries of the Sprudel, and the common origin of the springs has hereby been demonstrated in an unpleasant manner by the temporary disappearance of some other springs. Then the despicable little Tepl, which under ordinary circumstances is more aggravating on account of a deficiency rather than a surplus of water, has occasionally swelled up and destroyed human life, or at least much property —which latter event happened in a very alarming manner the last time in Nov., 1890. A historian of Carlsbad cannot pass over the calamity of 1865, when an insect, very small but very obnoxious, appeared in immense crowds and threatened to destroy the magnificent woods around Carlsbad. Man was powerless against it until in 1873 a saving angel at last appeared in the form of a diminutive spider, which also invaded the neighborhood in numberless crowds and devoured the insects to the "last man."—Some decennies ago Carlsbad still showed few outward traces of its high rank as a curing place. But the last few years have brought about great changes. Handsome city divisions, with modern houses, broad streets, and beautiful parks have arisen, monumental buildings have been erected over the springs, bath houses constructed, etc., etc. In these present days a plan will be carried out to give the town an excellent sewerage-system, and it is but fair to acknowledge in all this the result of energetic and successful endeavors to make the place fully worthy of its great and splendid fame.

Prices and Money.

Persons can live cheaply, even very cheaply, in Carlsbad, if they will agree to live in a modest style. But the celebrated Bohemian village is in general an expensive place—as everybody might expect in the very first health-resort on earth, open only five months a year, and situated in Austria, which is an expensive country. The lodgings are the dearest of all the visitors' necessities, and the prices in the most fashionable places in the height of the season are very high ; they vary very much, however, and are cheap during the early spring and autumn. The food is also tolerably dear. Then the tipping or "trinkgeld" system is very much developed, which sometimes rather disgusts visitors, especially the Americans, who are much less accustomed to it than the Europeans. I do not intend to defend the system—I think, indeed, that it is scarcely to be defended from any point of view, theoretical, moral, or practical,—but it is one of those things which the individual must take as they are and cannot change without injustice to others and unpleasant consequences to himself. Some necessities of life are cheap, *e. g.*, all articles for the toilet, clothes and boots, etc. Some articles of luxury are also to be had at low prices ; glass, earthenware, and china, and especially laces and embroideries are very cheap.

The money of Austria is at present as follows: Gulden or florin = 100 kreutzer. The gulden is equal to about forty-two American cents and to one English shilling and eight pence.

From 1893 gold will be introduced and the money will be the Krone = 100 heller = exactly 0.50 of the present gulden. A krone will thus be about 21 cents or 10 pence or very nearly equal to the French franc (which is about 20 cents).

Arrival in Carlsbad and Choice of Lodgings.

As soon as the visitor's baggage has been examined by the custom-house officers after his arrival at the depot,[1] he ought to take an " Einspänner " (carriage with one horse) or a " Zweispänner " (carriage with two horses)[2] and drive down to the

[1] The examination of the visitor's baggage is sometimes done at the frontier stations (Bodenbach, Eger), sometimes at the depot in Carlsbad, which is about a mile distant from those parts of the town wherein the visitor-patient generally takes up his quarters.

[2] The price for the " Einspänner " for persons and baggage is 1.50 fl., for the " Zweispänner " 2.50 fl.

town of Carlsbad, where his very first task will be
to take lodgings either for all of his stay or until
he has been able to make up his mind where he
wishes finally to settle. In order to arrange for
himself in the best possible way, the visitor must
remember the following rules and facts, which I
concentrate here in ten different paragraphs.

1. Never under any circumstances take rooms
which are offered at the depot.

2. All private houses in Carlsbad are lodging-
houses.

3. The visitor may, if he does not arrive
late at night, drive immediately to some of the
known parts of the town, *e. g.*, the Schlossberg, as
a starting-point for operations, and begin to look
about for rooms from the carriage. This task will
be facilitated by the " hausmeisters," or other
servants, who generally are to be found in the
streets, watching their opportunity of renting
rooms, and by the signs with the word "logis,"
which are put up in front of the houses as soon as
rooms are empty.

4. The visitor ought never to take any rooms
without seeing them himself and being thus able to
ascertain that they are airy, dry, and otherwise
healthy, and to decide if they suit him in point of
situation,[1] cleanliness, comfort, luxury, and price.

[1] For my own part I would prefer the heights and the outskirts of the town (the " Schlossberg," the " Hirschensprunggasse," the upper part of the " Parkstrasse," etc.) to the
lower and inner parts of it. But there are healthy and com-

The visitor must thoroughly make up his mind about those points *before* he takes the rooms *because—*

5. If the rooms are once taken (as the rule is) for an indefinite period, and even if this (as a rule) is done only by verbal agreement, the law (*i. e.*, " Miethesverordnung," § 9) presumes them to be taken for four weeks. If the visitor should wish to leave them before that time he must pay for two weeks after having stated his intention of leaving, *i. e.*, he must pay the whole week during which he leaves and another week besides. This too if he has slept only one night in the house; if he leaves it on the same day he has taken his apartment, he must pay for it for one week.

6. In the hotels the visitor can take his apartment only for the day, but ought distinctly and immediately on his arrival to state his intention of doing so and agree upon the price for the day.

7. The "American plan" of boarding, *i. e.*, paying a price which includes lodging and fare, whatever that fare may be, does not exist in Carlsbad. We always find there the "European plan," *i. e.*, you take your meals "à la carte" or, as the Americans sometimes very correctly put it, "you pay for what you eat."

8. The price for the apartment, and the price for the attendance (which last item is generally extra and amounts to one fl. to the "hausmeister" and one fortable rooms to be found all over Carlsbad—and taste differs.

fl. to the servant a week for every person, with some reduction for large parties), ought both to be distinctly and thoroughly agreed upon beforehand and understood by both parties. But I should dissuade visitors from requiring written contracts. The population is not accustomed to them, and they are unnecessary if only the verbal agreement is made *distinctly*.

9. The value of rooms varies according to the time of the season. If the visitor has taken his apartments for a definite period, the price cannot be altered during that period, and if for an indefinite period, the price cannot be altered for four weeks. But at the expiration of that term it can be altered. If a visitor takes an apartment for four weeks or for an indefinite period, *e. g.*, the 4th of May, he must prepare for an increased price if at the end of those four weeks he wishes to keep his apartments for a longer time. On the other hand, if he has taken his apartments, *e. g.*, on the 25th of July, for an indefinite period or for four weeks, he can, at the expiration of that time, lodge much cheaper either by insisting on a reduction of the former price or by removing to other quarters.

10. The visitor ought, as already stated, always himself to choose his lodgings. If he wishes to make this task easier, he may, some days before his arrival at Carlsbad, write a letter to his physician there,—spelling his physician's name correctly and writing his own name distinctly. The physician will then, either personally or by a letter left in his

office, on the visitor's arrival acquaint him where
eligible rooms may be had, and submit them to his
own choice. But rooms cannot be kept vacant for
anybody during the "season" at Carlsbad except
by paying for them from the day they are taken
in anybody's name.

6

Regulations Respecting Lodgings in Carlsbad.

1. Any stranger arriving in Carlsbad for the purpose of taking the waters is permitted to hire a lodging, either for a fixed or an indeterminate period of time.

As respects the rent itself, as well as the other details connected therewith, the written or oral contract, which may be concluded between the parties themselves, is considered as definite and binding.

2. If the lodging is hired for a fixed period, *i. e.*, for one, two, four, or six weeks, etc., or up to any fixed date, the contract so made shall be considered as in force during the whole of the time thus determined ; it does not require any notice of cessation, and when the period has run out it also expires, unless, by mutual agreement, a prolongation of the hiring shall be agreed upon, either under the same or other conditions, in which case, however, the prolongation is to be looked upon as a new contract.

3. The circumstance that the rent (as is usual in such cases) is paid by the week, has no influence whatever upon the contract.

4. During the continuance of hiring for a fixed period, the owner of the lodging cannot increase the rent to the tenant.

5. If the lodging be rented for an indefinite period, in cases of doubt, where no special contract shall have been entered into, it shall be assumed that the visitor has hired a lodging for the usual time of taking the waters, viz., four weeks ; and during this time no increase of the rent originally agreed upon may be attempted.

In the above case, if the hirer desires to quit his lodging at the end of the fourth week, or if the owner wishes to let it to some other person, it is necessary that a week's notice should be previously given. If this be not done, the contract runs on for a further indefinite time, and can then be put an end to at any time after a week's notice shall have been given.

6. If, however, the lodging is expressly rented by the week or by the day, then, in the first case a week's notice, and in the latter case a notice of twenty-four hours is necessary before leaving. The notice may be given either by the landlord or the tenant.

7. The week's notice commences with the last day of the week for which rent was last paid, and is to be reckoned from the day on which the liability for rent for the lodging was first incurred.

If notice be given to quit during the course of any week it will be regarded as having been given at the expiration of the week.

The week is reckoned as having seven days.

8. If, in the case of a lodging which is hired for an indefinite period or by the week, the lodger gives notice of his intention to leave during the first day he takes possession, he cannot be required to pay more than the rent for the current week.

9. If the lodger who has rented for an indefinite period or by the week desires to quit his lodging suddenly, he has not only to pay the rent for the current week, but also the amount of one additional week's rent as compensation in lieu of notice. At the same time he has no claim upon the lodging thus quitted, and has therefore no right to let it to any third person.

In the case of a lodging being hired by the day, the compensation to be paid is the amount of rent due for one day.

10. Every person letting lodgings has the right to demand from the hirer a deposit, which, however, shall not exceed the amount of one week's rent. This deposit is forfeited if the

hirer shall not take possession of the lodgings during the course of the first week, for which it is rented and does not furnish the owner with sufficient security that he is nevertheless willing to fulfil the terms of the contract. If he shall not furnish such a security the lodging-house keeper shall have the right at the termination of the week to let the lodging to any other person.

11. In hotels and boarding-houses strangers have a right to leave their apartments on any day and to pay only by the day. Should, however, a visitor hire a lodging in a hotel for a fixed price (not calculated by the day), whether it be for a fixed or indeterminate period, then the above regulations applicable to private houses come into force.

12. If the stipulations of the hiring contract are not kept by the lodging-house keeper, i. e., if the visitor shall not be provided with that which is contracted for, or is necessary ; if it can be shown that the lodging is dirty, damp, or in any way injurious to health ; or if faults shall be subsequently discovered which could not be ascertained at the time of hiring, whereby the lodger shall be disturbed in his rights of possession, and provided such faults can not be made good by the proprietor himself ;—in such cases the lodger shall have the right of leaving such lodging without any further notice or compensation other than paying for the actual time during which he remained in possession of the lodging.

13. In such a case the onus of proving the conditions which have been agreed to, as well as the faults complained of, shall lie with the lodger.

In the same way the onus of proof shall lie on the complainant if any dispute shall arise as to whether the lodging was hired for a fixed or indefinite period.

If no written contract be in existence between the parties, or the oral contract cannot be proved, then the *arrival sheet*, which contains a column for the period during which the visitor proposes to stay, shall be taken as proof ; and lodging-house keepers are advised to cause the **arrival sheet** to be

filled up by the visitors themselves ; as where this is not done
the assertion of the visitors must be taken as proof.

14. In the case of furnished lodgings no extra charge can
be made for injury or deterioration sustained by furniture,
beds, or other articles in the course of ordinary fair wear and
tear ; but

    a. In the case of anything being wilfully broken or
    damaged compensation must be paid.
    b. In case of severe or prolonged illness, when an un-
    usually large amount of bed linen is required, then a
    corresponding amount of compensation may be de-
    manded for the extra supply. In any case, when
    articles may be rendered unfit for use, the expense of
    replacing them may be charged for.

15. Every visitor has a right to procure his meals and his
food of all kinds, as well as his baths, where he pleases, and he
has also the right to have his washing done wherever it may
best suit him.

Any attempt to restrict these rights which may be imposed
upon the visitor at the time of renting the lodging has no legal
effect. The lodging-house keeper can base no right of action
thereupon, and, moreover, it entitles the hirer to repudiate the
contract without any further notice.

16. In the rent of the lodging the charge for attendance is
not usually considered to be included, unless it be proved that
the lodging was hired for this or that price, to include attendance. In any other case the charge for attendance shall be a
matter of mutual agreement, or shall be determined according
to the tariff usual in the house.

If, however, the charge for attendance be demanded according to a fixed tariff by the landlord or lodging-house keeper in
the usual weekly or monthly account, and shall be paid to him
by the lodger, the servants have no claim to a separate gratuity
and the stranger is under no obligation to pay them any such.

Moreover, under the term attendance is to be understood

the services usually called for, such as cleaning and putting in order of the rooms, carrying water or other necessaries, as well as other such small services as may be usual ; but the ironing of linen, washing, mending, and cleaning of clothes or of boots, or waiting upon the sick is expressly excluded.

17. Disputes arising out of any hiring contract are to be laid before the Royal District Assessor in the Amtsgebäude (District Office), 2d floor, Neue Wiese, who shall take the matter in hand as arbitrator and endeavor to arrange matters by means of a mutual understanding ; but in case he shall not be successful in effecting this, he shall then direct the parties to apply to the law courts.

If both parties to the dispute shall agree thereto, the District Assessor may be called upon to give a judicial decision in the matter.

Hotels in Carlsbad.

Grand Hotel Pupp (with dependencies), in the southern end of the town in the valley, but close to the woods. A very fashionable and splendid establishment with about 400 rooms, good restaurant, frequent musical entertainments, and with every modern accommodation.

Hotel Bristol (with dependencies), in the most magnificent situation on the Schlossberg, surrounded by its own grounds, overlooking the valley of the Eger and the mountains. A good hotel with every comfort—the Hotel Bristol forms, with the beautiful **Königsvilla** (independent), and the **Villa Teresa** and with the neighboring villas on the Schlossberg, the headquarters of the Anglo-American visitors.

Hotel Anger (Neue Wiese).

Hotel Continental (Marktplatz).

Hotel Goldener Schild and Zwei deutsche Monarchen (Neue Wiese).

Hotel Kroh or **Donau** (Parkstrasse)

Hotel Hannover (Markt).

Hotel Russie }
"   Morgenstern } (Kaiserstrasse).
"   Royal }
Hotel Hopfenstock }
"   Rheinischer Hof } (Geweihdiggasse).
"   Loib }
Hotel National (Gartenzeile).
Hotel Poste }
"   Bayrischer Hof } (Egerstrasse).
Hotel Fassmann }
"   Lyon }
"   Bellevue } (Bahnhofstrasse).
"   Stadt Schneeberg }
Hotel Drei Fasanen (Kirchengasse).
Glattauers Hotel (Parkstrasse. In this hotel table according to Jewish rites).

Cook's Agency in Carlsbad

is held by the well-known banking-firm **Gottfried Lederer,** from whom the visitors in Carlsbad can receive any necessary information about their journeys (in English or in a dozen other languages), and may buy their travelling tickets to any part of the world. The locality is in the "Ritter" house, near where the Mühlbadgasse opens upon the Markt, opposite the Marktbrunnen.

Banks and Exchanges.

The above-named Cook's agent **Lederer,** in Mühlbadgasse, **Benedikt** in the "Alte Wiese" and on the corner of the Stadthaus, the **Bohemian Escompte-Bank** in the Mühlbadgasse, **Schwalb** in the Markt and in the Alte Wiese.

Post, Telegraph, and Custom-House

is to be found in the "Markt," open from 7 A.M. until midnight. The visitor will leave his address in the post-office and will then get his mail sent to his home three times a day.

Postage stamps are to be had at the following places, in the immediate neighborhood of which post-boxes are placed :

Moritz Ehrlich, "Kaiser von Oesterreich," Mühlbadgasse ; Wilhelm Rispler, "zum Matrosen,"and "zum blauen Schiff" Neue Wiese ; Heinrich Eberhart, "Erzherzogin Sophie," Marienbaderstrasse ; Anton Neubauer, "Erfurt," Schulgasse ; S. Rosenfeld's Sohn, Stadt "Wiesbaden," Sprudelgasse ; Anton Sebert's Witwe, "Nordisches Haus," Kreuzgasse ; L. Löwenstein, "zum Italiener," Pragergasse ; Gebrüder Mosauer, Bahnhofstrasse ; Fanni Obergruper, k. k. Tabaktrafikantin, "Rosenthal," Egerstrasse ; Lotti Neubauer, Pragergasse, Omnibus-Aufnahms-Lokale "zum goldenen Schild" ; Hermine Eckert, "Britannia."

Mayer's Tourist Office

in the "Savoyen" house, Alte Wiese, sells tickets, sends luggage, etc.

Ulrich and Gross' Luggage Expedition

in the "Goldene Löwe" house, Kaiserstrasse.

Churches.

In the **English (Anglican)** Church, on the Schlossberg, divine service is held at 11 A.M. and 4 P.M. on Sundays.

In the **Roman-Catholic** Cathedral masses are held daily at 7, at 9, and at 10 A.M. On Sundays at 7 and at 8 A.M. masses, sermon after the mass at 10 A.M., at 11 A.M. mass.

In the **Protestant** Church there is a sermon at 11 A.M. on Sundays.

In the **Russian** Church (Marienbaderstrasse) service is held at 11 A.M. on Sundays.

In the **Synagogue** (Parkstrasse) morning and evening service is held daily, and, besides this, on the Sabbath is held thora and mussaph service at 10 A.M. and another service at 3 P.M.

Music.

Labitzsky's orchestra plays from 4–6 P.M. on Sundays in the Stadtpark (free). On Tuesdays and Thursdays at Pupp's establishment (free).

An orchestra also plays from 7.30–9 P.M. On Mondays and Fridays in the Stadtpark (free). On Wednesdays at Pupp's establishment (free).

An orchestra also plays from 4–6 P.M. (entrance, 0. 50 fl.) on Mondays at the Café Posthof, on Wednesdays at Café Schönbrunn, on Fridays at the Café Posthof (Symphonies).

An orchestra plays from 6–8 A.M. every day at the Mühlbrunnen and the Sprudel.

Stadt-Theater (Neue Wiese).

A beautiful little theatre ; it usually gives representations every evening during the season. The best places cost 2 fl.

Apothecaries' Stores.

" Zum weissen Adler " Markt (Herr Worlicek).
" Kronen-Apotheke" Mühlbrunnen (Herr Lippman).

Mattonis Mineral-Water Store

in the house " Mercur " on the Markt, offers all kinds of mineral waters and their products.

The Carlsbad-Water for Exportation

and its products sold by Loebel & Schottländer, Egerstrasse
575. The "Sprudelsalzwerk" is to be seen from 10–12 daily
in No. 720 Morgenzeile.

The Burgomaster's (Mayor's) and the Police-Office

is in the Stadthaus, Mühlbadgasse, opposite and quite near to
the Mühlbrunnen. This is the place to report about lost or
found articles, to retrieve against an unjust taxation in the
" Kur- und Music-Taxe," and to complain against wrongs
from any person whatever.

Bezirkhauptmannschaft,

where legal questions arising between visitors and inhabitants
in Carlsbad are decided, is Neue Wiese 578 (on the other side
the Tepl, opposite Alte Wiese and not far from Pupp's establishment).

Tariff for the Baths.

Mineral-"Salon"-bath, A.M. or P.M..................Fl1.60	
Mineral bath until 2 P.M..........................	1.10
" " after "	0.80
Mineral douche-bath..............................	1.60
Russian vapor-bath with cold douche but without attendance.....................................	1.00
Cold douche without attendance....................	0.60
Mud-bath with cleaning bath......................	2.10
"Salon" mud-bath.................................	3.10
Mud foot-bath, A.M., with linen...................	1.72
" " " without......................	1.58

Mud foot-bath, P.M., without......................	1.28
Mud-bath for the arm, A.M........................	1.48
" " P.M........................	1.04
(Neubad) mud-" Salon "-bath......................	3.10
Steel bath (Eisenbad)........	1.00
Acidulous bath (Sauerbrunnen).....................	1.00
Sweet-water-bath (Süsswasserbad)..................	1.00
" Kommunebad " (Don't go there !)................	0.05
Heating the bathing cabinet.......................	0.20
Bathing-robe (Bademantel)	0.20
Bathing-sheet (Leintuch)..........................	0.10
Towel (Handtuch)................................	0.04
Mud (6 kilo).....................................	0.24
Sprudelsoap for a bath............................	0.70
Sea salt 1 kilo	0.40
Common salt 1 kilo...............................	0.20

The "Kurtaxe"

or what every visitor (whether he uses the water or not) must
pay after eight days' stay in Carlsbad is (for the whole cure):

For rich persons (First Class)......................	10 fl.
For persons of means (Second Class)................	6 "
For persons of small means (Third Class)............	4 "
Children under fourteen and servants (Fourth Class)....	1 "

The visitor need not trouble himself as to where he shall
pay this tax, a collector will always come for the money, and
at the same time will also collect the

"Musiktaxe"

which the visitors also pay according to their different classes,
so that the first class pays for a party of 1, 2, 3, 4, or 5 persons
5, 8, 11, 14, or 17 florins, the second class pays the analogous

prices of 3, 5, 6, 7, or 8 florins, the third class 2, 3, 4, 5, or 6 florins. Physicians or Austrian officers pay for themselves and families 2 or 3 florins. Only people with a certificate of poverty are free from paying this tax.

Tariff for Carriages.

	1 horse	2 horses
	" Einspänner "	" Zweispänner "
I. From the railway station to any point of the city, or *vice versa*.....	1.20 fl.	2.00 fl.
The same way from 9 P.M. to 6 A.M..	1.50	2.50
For any delay in the city each 30 minutes.........................	0.40	0.60
For heavier luggage................	0.30	0.50
II. In Carlsbad		
For the first 15 minutes...........	0.50	—
" " 30 "	0.80	1.20
For each succeeding quarter of an hour	0.20	
" " half "	—	0.60
III. From any point in Carlsbad for going to		
Sans Souci, Schönbrunn, Posthof..	0.70	1.00
Drahowitz, Freundschaftsaal Kaiserpark, Jägerhaus, and Friedhof.....	1.20	1.80
Restaurant Leibold in Pirkenhammer	1.50	2.20
Setlitz, Schwarzenbergbrücke, Aich, Dallwitz, Fischern, Pirkenhammer	2.00	3.00
Altrolau, Aberg, Leonard, Bergwirthshaus.........................	2.60	4.00
For the return is to pay [for the waiting and the time spent in returning] every half hour.................	0.40	0.60
IV. For going from and returning to any point of Carlsbad and for a maximum waiting time of three hours.		
Schlackenwerth, Lichtenstadt, Tippelsgrün, Engelhaus............	4.50	6.70

	1 horse	2 horses
	" Einspänner "	" Zweispänner "
Elbogen, Giesshübl-Puchstein, Giesshübl (Factory)	5.00	8.00
Petschau	6.00	9.00
Joachimsthal	7.00	10.00
Over Pirkenhammer to Aich and back	4.00	6.00
To St. Leonhard and back through Aich	4.00	6.00
St. Leonard, Aberg, Esterhazyweg, Pirkenhammer, Carlsbad	4.00	6.00
Zettlitz, Altrolau, Donitz, Carlsbad	4.00	6.00
Fischern, Putschirn, Kellerberg, Altrolau, Carlsbad	4.60	7.00
Pirkenhammer, Funkenstein (Metzeryhöhe), Carlsbad	5.00	8.00
Schlackenwerth, Lichtenstadt, Carlsbad	6.00	9.00
Funkenstein, Schneidmühl, Pirkenhammer, Carlsbad	6.00	9.00
Fischern, Altrolau, Tippelsgrün, Lichtenstadt, Carlsbad	6.00	9.00
Elbogen (waiting at), Hans Heiling, Aich, Carlsbad	6.00	9.00
Pirkenhammmer, Funkenstein, Kohlau, Schneidmuhl, Espenthor, Carlsbad	6.00	9.00
The last trip, including Engelhaus, Elbogen, Schlaggenwald, Pirkenhammer, Carlsbad	7.00	10.00
Giesshübl (with or without) Schlackenwerth, Carlsbad	7.00	10.00
Giesshübl (with or without) Schlackenwerth, Carlsbad	7.00	10.00

Omnibus-Cars and their Tariffs.

To and from the Depot.

A car starts from the Theaterplatz about an hour before the departure of every train. For every person is paid 40 kr. ; for baggage on the roof of the car 10 kr. a piece.

To and from Pirkenhammer (China-Factory).

From Carlsbad (Theaterplatz).	Arrival at the Restaurant Leibold in Pirkenhammer.	Arrival at the China-Factory in Pirkenhammer.
1.30 P.M.	2.00 P.M.	2.10 P.M.
2.00 "	2.30 "	2.40 "
3.00 "	3.30 "	3.40 "
3.30 "	4.00 "	4.10 "

Departure from the China-Factory.

2.10 P.M.	2.40 P.M.	3.40 P.M.	4.10 P.M.	5.10 P.M.

Departure from the Restaurant Leibold.

12.30 P.M.	2.50 P.M.	6.00 P.M.
1.00 "	5.00 "	6.30 "
2.25 "	5.30 "	7.00 "

Every person pays 40 kr.

To and from Aich (China-Factory).

From Theaterplatz, 1.45 P.M. and 3.30 P.M.
From Aich, 12.45 P.M., 2.45 P.M., 5.45 P.M.
Every person pays 40 kr.

To and from Fischern (China-Factory).

The car starts from Kaiserstrasse, opposite the Felsenquelle ; tickets are to be had in the Ulrich & Gross office (Goldene Löwe.")

From Carlsbad, 2.30 and 3.30 P.M.

From the China-Factory in Fischern, 6 and 7 P.M.   Price 30 kr.

To and from Dallwitz (China Factory).

The car starts from Becherplatz, 1.30 P.M. and 3.30 P.M. ; returns to Carlsbad, 5.30 and 7.30 P.M.   Price 50 kr.

To and from Giesshübl-Puchstein.

Tickets are sold in Mattoni's office, house " Merkur " in the Marktplatz.   The car starts 11 A.M., and 1 P.M. from the Theaterplatz, and returns from Giesshübl at 6 P.M.   The whole trip costs 1.50 fl.

To and from Joachimsthal and Keilberg.

Tickets are bought in Otto Blayer's office, in the house " Kaiserkrone " in the Kaiserstrasse.   The car starts 9 A.M. from the Kaiserstrasse, opposite the Felsenquelle, and returns at 8 P.M.   The whole trip costs 3 fl.

Tariff for the Donkey-Carriages and for the Riding-Donkeys.

Tickets are bought in the Stadthaus at the Stadtkasse in the Mühlbadgasse.

For the whole day............................4.50 fl.
For the whole day, if hired per week........... 4.00 "
For the half day............................. 3.00 "
For a trip to the Kreuzberg or the Hircshensprung
    in the forenoon, or to any place at the same
    distance............................... 1.50 "
For a ride or drive on level ground in the fore-
    noon, per hour........................... 0.80 "

For a drive to, or to and from, any of the bathing-
houses in the forenoon................... 0.80 fl.

Tariff for Rolling-Chairs and for Express-
men.

Rolling-chair with attendance, for one hour...... 0.70 fl.
Rolling-chair with attendance during several hours,
   per hour.............................. 0.50 "
For an expressman within the town and with lighter weight
than 15 kilo. :

¼ hour.	½ hour.	1 hour.	Every hour afterwards.
0.15 fl.	0.20 fl.	0.30 fl.	0.15 fl.

For an expressman outside the town, or with heavier weight
or harder work

¼ hour.	½ hour.	1 hour.	Every hour afterwards.
0.20 fl.	0.30 fl.	0.40 fl.	0.20 fl.

Between 9 P.M. and 6 A.M. the prices of the expressmen are
increased by 50 per cent.

Excursions.*

Puppsche Allée—Kiesweg—Posthof—Freundschaftsaal
—Kaiserpark.

This is the most frequented walk outside the precincts of
the town. You start from Pupp's establishment, following
the whole time the left bank of the (at this point) limpid Tepl,
passing the restaurant **Sans Souci,** then the **Kiesweg** with
its many booths and shops, and the **Erzherzog-Karls-
Brücke** (without crossing it). After this the walk follows the

* To understand these short notes the reader had better buy
a map of Carlsbad, which may be had at the booksellers for
ten kr.

broad **Marienbaderstrasse**, and successively takes you by the restaurants **Posthof** and **Freundschaftsaal**, till you arrive, after half an hour's walk, at the restaurant **Kaiserpark**. From this place you may return to town :

1. By crossing the Tepl at Kaiserpark, and by following the **Schwindelweg** on the **Plobenberg** to Schönbrunn, whence, by recrossing the Tepl, you find yourself again in the Marienbaderstrasse near the Kiesweg.

2. Or by returning the same way you came to a place between the Kaiserpark and the Freundschaftsaal, and by then taking the **Faulenzerweg** over the hills ; you will then, after having passed the **Ecce-Homo Chapel** and the **Findlaters Tempel**, reach the southern part of Carlsbad.

3. Or by returning the same way as far as the Posthof and leaving the Marienbaderstrasse on your right, and passing the **Schwarzenberg-Denkmal**, take the **Vier-Uhr Promenade** down to Kiesweg.

Dorotheenau — Sauerbrunnen—Schweitzerhof—Schönbrunn.

The right bank of the Tepl in the southern neighborhood of the Erzherzog-Karls-Brücke is called **Dorotheenau**. We find in the immediate vicinity and within sight the two coffeehouses **Schweitzerhof** and **Schönbrunn**, the "**Sauerbrunnen**," with its bathing-house and the **Stephaniequelle**.

Hammer or Pirkenhammer

is a village with a [very well worth seeing] china-factory. It will take you about an hour to walk to the place ; the road is the same as the one to the Kaiserpark—you there take the Marienbaderstrasse and cross the Tepl, having Pirkenhammer in sight as soon as you have passed Kaiserpark.

A car starts several times a day from the Theaterplatz for Pirkenhammer (see p. 94). The carriages have a tariff for

7

going to the place. There are two coffee-houses, **Leibold** and **Habsburg.**

Hirschensprung

is a rock westward of the Marktplatz, and quite near to and visible from many parts of the town. You may reach it by taking a little road which passes up from the house " Zur Zufriedenheit " in the **Hirschensprunggasse,** or by taking the road from the English Church up to the Jägerhaus, and leaving it when a sign on the left hand indicates the smaller road to the Hirschensprung.

Ecce-Homo-Kapelle—Findlaters Tempel—Franz-Joseph's Höhe—Belvedere—Friedrich-Wilhelm-Platz, etc.,

are all found in the western neighborhood of the town where the beautiful forest-covered hills are intersected by many miles of pleasant roads (Neue-Weg, Choteksche-Weg, Bontourlinweg, etc., etc.).—The terminus for a walk in this district is often the

Aberg,

a promontory (with a restaurant and a belvedere) about two English miles southwest of Carlsbad ; the whole trip will take the better part of the forenoon or afternoon. The most beautiful way is from the **Jägerhaus** (not far from the English church) over the **Bild,** a place in the midst of the woods for Roman Catholic devotion with an image of the Holy Virgin.

The best way to return is along the little road down to **St. Leonhard,** passing thereafter the **Echo** and reaching Carlsbad either over the **Jägerhaus** or the **Schweitzerthal** or the **Marien-Sophien-Weg,** which last road leads to the northern part of the town.

Persons to whom walking the whole way would be somewhat fatiguing can make the trip in a donkey car.

Stephanplatz — Panorama — Camera Obscura — Drei-kreutzberg—König-Otto-Höhe—Ewiges Leben and Stephaniewarte

are all in view of Carlsbad on the heights of the right side of the Tepl. Starting from the cathedral by the **Schulgasse** you reach the Stephanplatz-terrace (in its vicinity is the **Panorama** Restaurant, with a fine view), and some minutes' walk to the Northeast from this place is the **"Camera Obscura"** with a still finer view. A small road from the Camera takes you in a Southwestern direction successively to the top of the three heights, **Dreikreutzberg** (335 metres), **König-Otto-Höhe** (578 m.) and **Ewiges Leben** (636 m.) with a belvedere, the **Stephaniewarte**. From this place you may descend to and reach Carlsbad through the **Pragerstrasse**. The trip takes a whole forenoon or afternoon.

Wiesenthal,

with its chalybeate spring and its bathing-house is directly north of the Stadtpark some few minutes distant. A half an hours' walk leisurely eastward from this place will bring you to the village **Drahowitz** with its chalybeate spring (the "Rothe Säuerling").

Dallwitz

is a village with a china-factory and a castle about an hour's walk north of Carlsbad. The purpose of the trip is generally to see the factory and the mighty oak in the park ("Körner's Eiche") Restaurant "Zu drei Eichen."

(Concerning the car see p. 95 and concerning the tariff for carriages p. 92).

Giesshübl-Puchstein

is a little watering-place 1½ hours' drive northeast of Carlsbad, chiefly known on account of the celebrated mineral water Giesshübler, which flows up from the rock above the place.

No person visiting Carlsbad for any considerable length of time ought to omit seeing this place, both on account of its own merits, and on account of the beautiful drive thither. One starts from Carlsbad conveniently at 11 A.M. and takes dinner at Giesshübl, or one starts from Carlsbad at 4 P.M. and returns after having taken supper at Giesshübl.

Engelhaus

are the ruins, on the top of a rock (about four English miles eastward from Carlsbad), of a very old castle which appears in history in the fourteenth century and may have been old even at that period. It shared the fate of so many other strongholds in Bohemia : of being taken and destroyed during the thirty years' war by the Swedes. A village at the foot of the rock.

(Concerning the tariff for carriages see p. 92.)

Aich—Hans Heiling—Elbogen.

Aich is a village (with about 3000 inhabitants) about 1½ English miles west of Carlsbad. There are a china factory and an old castle ; the latter, which overlooks the river Eger, has been turned into a restaurant.

Hans Heiling is an exceedingly romantic place, (celebrated in many tales, ballads, poems, and an opera), about half an hour's walk along the right bank of the Eger southwest of Aich. There is a small restaurant, where one often has opportunities of observing typical German life.

Elbogen is a town (3500 inh.) some miles southwest of Carlsbad, whence it can be reached in three hours on foot, in one hour and a half by driving, and in about an hour by rail. It is a beautiful place, and the castle (now a prison) is about a thousand years old and well worth seeing.

The best way to see all three of these places is to start for Elbogen at about 11 A.M. in a carriage (see p. 93), to take dinner on the terrace above the Eger at the restaurant

" Weisses Ross," to walk leisurely (in about an hour) to Hans Heiling, thence to go down the river in a boat to Aich, where the carriage, sent back for this purpose from Elbogen, will be waiting at the landing place.

Joachimsthal—Gottesgab—Sonnenwirbel.

Joachimsthal in the Erzgebirge, 2½ hour's drive from Carlsbad, is a town of 7000 inhabitants, 2000 of whom are employed in the mines (chiefly iron, but also silver, kobalt, nickel, lead, and uranium). A great cigar-factory gives employment to 700 persons. The women are chiefly occupied in making laces (which are sold at fabulously cheap prices in Carlsbad). An hour's drive from Joachimsthal carries us still farther upward to the little town of **Gottesgab,** in whose vicinity we may ascend the mount **Sonnenwirbel** (1232 metres) with a fine view over parts of Bohemia and Saxony. It is best to leave Carlsbad after breakfast, to proceed through Joachimsthal to Gottesgab, but order dinner in the first place, which will then be ready when you return from Gottesgab. The tariff only determines the price to Joachimsthal (resp. 7 or 10 fl.)—a special agreement must be made for the trip to Gottesgab.

THE END.

www.ingramcontent.com/pod-product-compliance
Lightning Source LLC
Chambersburg PA
CBHW030545270326
41927CB00008B/1520